Introduction to Teaching and Learning in Health Professions

FIRST AUSTRALIAN AND NEW ZEALAND EDITION

Introduction to Teaching and Learning in Health Professions

FIRST AUSTRALIAN AND NEW ZEALAND EDITION

Dr Lisa McKenna PhD MEdSt RN RM
Professor
Faculty of Medicine, Nursing and Health Sciences
Monash University, Melbourne

Dr Lynette Stockhausen PhD MEdSt BEd DipTeach RN
Associate Professor
School of Health and Human Sciences
Southern Cross University, Gold Coast

Wolters Kluwer | Lippincott Williams & Wilkins

Senior Acquisitions Editor: Penny Martin
Product Manager: Jacqueline Johnson
Editor: Karen Enkelaar, Do Write
Indexer: Puddingburn Publishing Services
Typesetter: Midland Typesetters, Australia
Cover design: Kim Webber
Printer: McPhersons Printing Group

National Library of Australia Cataloguing-in-Publication entry
Author: Lisa McKenna and Lynette Stockhausen
Title: Introduction to Teaching and Learning in Health Professions
Edition: first edition
ISBN: 9781920994525
Dewey number: 610.7
Subjects: Clinical medicine—Study and teaching/Medical logic—Study and teaching/Patients—
Care—Study and teaching/Medical personnel and patient—Study and teaching.

Contents

Preface

Many health professional standards now incorporate teaching roles and responsibilities. Within the context of an increasing complexity of client care, needs and management, health professionals are required to play a greater role in teaching students and peers. This role is often undertaken concurrently while conducting client care and responsibilities.

Despite the teaching role being explicit within professional standards for some health professions, it is frequently presumed that individuals can automatically assume this role. Often this is not different for health professionals who choose to enter academia. There are few simple and handy resources available to assist professionals in carrying out such educational roles. With this in mind, we felt a need to develop a resource to support health professionals, particularly those new to such roles, when assuming their teaching roles and developing expertise. We view this book as an introduction to entering into such roles on which further learning may be developed.

In addition, to support and guide health professionals in acquiring educational roles, this book will be useful to a range of students across the health professions. This includes undergraduate students who are expected to demonstrate achievement of teaching-related professional competencies prior to graduation, as well as postgraduate students undertaking education courses with a focus on health professions.

The book is divided into four sections, outlined in the following pages. Each chapter, within each section, presents the reader with theoretical perspectives on teaching and learning and provides practical tips and exercises for active learning. While the various health professions may conduct their curricula in slightly different ways, this book is presented so as to accommodate these variations.

Section One: Overview of Education in the Health Professions

This section provides the reader with an overview of education in the health professions, including how it fits within the larger academic curriculum and the settings where education occurs. In Chapter 1, *Locating Education in the Health Professions,* we examine the goals and underpinnings of teaching, teaching roles often used in the health professions, and contexts for health professional education.

Section Two: Foundations for Supporting Learning

The second section provides an overview of factors that need to be considered in effective health professional education, including recognising diversity among the student population, learning styles and complexities of the teaching settings (including multidisciplinary approaches and current constraints). In Chapter 2, *Learners in the Health Professions,* we explore who the learners are in the health professions, and address their learning needs by examining theories underpinning learning, such as adult learning theory. We examine critical thinking and supporting learning. In Chapter 3, *Situated Learning and Learning Communities*, we consider learning in the workplace, social and political influences on learning in these contexts, and professional socialisation.

Section Three: Creating Optimal Learning Environments

In the third section the reader is led through the practical cycle of teaching, from preparation through to practice to evaluation. It provides practical and realistic strategies for optimising the learning experience. Chapter 4, *Preparation for Learning*, presents a range of strategies needed for successful teaching and learning, such as lesson planning, the development of learning outcome statements, and relationship building. In Chapter 5, *Constructing Learning*, we explore the practicalities of putting the planning into action. The chapter introduces different types of teaching approaches and how to facilitate meaningful learning. Chapter 6, *Transforming Learning*, builds further on the previous chapter by expanding on effective methods for teaching and learning. *Reflection and Reconstruction*, Chapter 7, covers the important areas of optimising learning outcomes through promotion of reflective practice, and constructive feedback and assessment of learning.

Section Four: Developing Teaching and Learning

The final section provides scope for the reader to develop expertise in, and strategies for, managing commonly encountered situations in health professional teaching. Furthermore, it presents strategies for ongoing development of the teacher. Chapter 8, *Challenging Student Situations*, presents examples of situations that can occur within practice settings that teachers may encounter and how these can be sensitively and appropriately managed to impact positively on learning. Finally, Chapter 9, *Developing as a Teacher*, discusses strategies by which health professionals can develop expertise in their teaching roles.

Resources

We encourage readers to develop their repertoire of skills, knowledge and attitudes around learning and teaching, regardless of the setting. The resources section at the end of the book is designed as a 'toolkit' to assist with effectively managing the practicalities of day-to-day teaching and learning.

To inform the content throughout the book, we draw on our own extensive research and academic and clinical teaching experiences. We hope all users will find it a beneficial addition to their professional libraries and teacher development.

Lisa McKenna and Lynette Stockhausen

About the Authors

Dr Lisa McKenna PhD MEdSt RN RM
Lisa McKenna has over 20 years of experience in academia and is currently a Professor at Monash University in Melbourne, Australia. She has previously held senior education roles within the Faculty of Medicine, Nursing and Health Sciences and School of Nursing and Midwifery at Monash.

Lisa has both a national and international reputation in health professional education. She has worked extensively in classroom environments and clinical education settings, and she has had heavy engagement in curriculum development. In 2012, Lisa received a Vice Chancellor's Award for Programs that Enhance Learning at Monash University and one of her textbooks received an Australian Educational Publishing Award.

Lisa's research has explored a range of aspects relating to the education of health professionals. This research has predominantly focused on practice-based learning, students' development of their professional roles and attributes, graduate transition to practice, peer teaching and learning, and interprofessional education.

Dr Lynette Stockhausen PhD MEdSt BEd DipTeach RN
Lynette Stockhausen has had 30 years of experience as an academic in a number of universities throughout Australia. She has held professorial and leadership positions, ensuring best practices and continuous improvement in teaching and learning.

Lynette has a national and international profile in health professional education. In particular, she has worked extensively in clinical education and curriculum development. Lynette has undertaken education consultancies in the United Kingdom, Singapore, Vietnam, New Zealand and Japan. In 2002, Lynette was a World Health Organisation Official to Vietnam, where she assisted in the development and writing of the Vietnamese Nursing Standards in line with the International Council of Nurses Guidelines. She also conducted clinical teaching workshops for health and education departments.

Lynette's research has concentrated on the exploration of the unique learning that occurs in workplace settings and pedagogical approaches to educational technologies.

Reviewers

Joe Acker DipHSc(cand) MA(Lead) GradCert(T&L High Ed)
    HonDip(paramed) MPA
Senior Lecturer & Paramedic Program Leader
School of Biomedical Science, Faculty of Science
Charles Sturt University, Port Macquarie, New South Wales

Melanie Birks PhD RN BN
Professor
School of Nursing and Midwifery
Central Queensland University, Noosa, Queensland

Ted Brown PhD MSc MPA BScOT(Hons) GradCert(HPE) OT(C) OT(R)
Associate Professor, Postgraduate Coordinator & Undergraduate
    Program Convenor
Department of Occupational Therapy, School of Primary Health
    Care, Faculty of Medicine, Nursing and Health Science
Monash University, Frankston, Victoria

Clare Cole BN GradCertNurs(Ortho) MEdSt
Lecturer/Academic
School of Health Sciences (Nursing)
University of Ballarat, Mt Helen, Victoria

Les Fitzgerald RN RM DipTeachNurs BEd MNursSt PhD
Head, Department of Rural Nursing & Midwifery
La Trobe Rural Health School
La Trobe University, Bendigo, Victoria

Melanie Greenwood MN GradCert(T&L High Ed) Cert(IC)
    Cert(NeuroSc)
Senior Lecturer, Coordinator Postgraduate Studies
School of Nursing and Midwifery
University of Tasmania, Hobart, Tasmania

Tania Johnston BScN MHSt(Lead)
Lecturer, Paramedic Programs
School of Biomedical Sciences
Charles Sturt University, Port Macquarie, New South Wales

Bill Lord BHSc(PreHospCare) GradDip(CBL) MEd PhD
Associate Professor
Paramedic Science, School of Health and Sport Sciences
University of the Sunshine Coast, Maroochydore, Queensland

Tamara Page BN MNSc
Lecturer and Course Coordinator for Master Clinical Nursing
School of Nursing, Faculty of Health Sciences
University of Adelaide, Adelaide, South Australia

Wendy Penney RN MN PhD
Discipline Head Nursing
School of Health Science
University of Ballarat, Ballarat, Victoria

Bodil Rasmussen RN MEdSt PhD FACN
Senior Lecturer
School of Nursing and Midwifery, Faculty of Health
Deakin University, Burwood, Victoria

Maree Donna Simpson BPharm BSc(Hons) PhD MPS
GradCert(T&L High Ed)
Associate Professor
School of Biomedical Sciences
Charles Sturt University, Orange, New South Wales

Acknowledgements

For a number of years, we have being working towards publishing this book, driven by our passion for education and for providing quality learning experiences for learners. However, this book would not have been possible without the input of many people.

We are extremely grateful to the many reviewers who provided us with invaluable feedback, and who assisted us in strengthening the final product.

We are incredibly thankful to Penny Martin and Jackie Johnson from Lippincott Williams & Wilkins for their ongoing encouragement, guidance and support throughout all stages of the book's development, along with all those involved in its production.

Finally, we are especially grateful to our respective families: Hayley, Lachlan and Gerald, and Nobby, for their patience, support and encouragement throughout the development of this book.

Lisa McKenna and Lynette Stockhausen

Overview of Education in the Health Professions

CHAPTER 1

Locating Education in the Health Professions

KEY CONCEPTS
- Education underpinnings
- Goals of teaching
- Bridging theory and practice
- Clinical competence
- Teaching roles for health professionals
- Clinical teaching contexts
- Delivering education
  - The classroom
  - Clinical placements
- Teaching relationships and models
- Challenges in classroom and clinical settings

INTRODUCTION

Education is fundamental to the development of professional expertise across health professional courses. Teaching environments include traditional lectures and tutorials, or clinical laboratories and clinics, depending on the actual profession. Learning experiences in clinical settings are often extensively interwoven throughout the educational curricula. Clinical, or fieldwork, placements have the potential to impact on students' career choices, areas for later practice specialisation and, for some, even whether to continue in their chosen health profession. In addition, they have a role to play in future healthcare workforce recruitment and retention. The clinical placement experience forms a significant component in preparatory educational programs for health professionals. It allows for the application of classroom learning and the development of expertise in a range of professional areas. As part of the overall educational program, learning during each placement (or practicum) is designed to develop related classroom learning and professional practice.

This chapter introduces the area of education in the health professions. It particularly examines the place of clinical education and its position within the larger academic curriculum. It examines where education occurs, who provides the teaching, and models by which that teaching is delivered. Across the different health professions, language around the area of clinical education varies significantly. Within this book we have chosen to use the broad term 'practice partner' to describe a person who, on a day-to-day basis, provides direct client care or services while simultaneously facilitates learning and professional development in the practice setting. Later in this chapter we explore different models used for the provision of clinical education, and unpack different specific terminology used to refer to those who teach in clinical settings.

EDUCATION UNDERPINNINGS

Before we can explore concepts surrounding teaching, it is important to establish contexts surrounding the provision of education and where the health professional educator fits into this.

ACADEMIC CURRICULUM

The academic curriculum constitutes all of the theoretical and practical learning required for a student to successfully complete their course; hence, it consists of both classroom and clinical learning. In most health professions, the academic curriculum requires accreditation by relevant professional bodies to ensure that graduates are able to register to practice. Professional bodies often prescribe particular requirements for academic programs, such as minimum numbers of clinical hours, or the inclusion of specific content such as Indigenous health.

CLINICAL CURRICULUM

Clinical education constitutes an important role in the education of health professionals. It is easy, though, to take a simplistic view of this part of the educational process by seeing it as just practising skills learnt in the classroom. Clinical education is a component of the larger, more complex academic curriculum. It is designed to build upon classroom theory and allow for the application of knowledge-into-practice contexts. Thus each clinical learning experience is guided by specific learning outcomes that are expected to be achieved within an allocated time. However, while we may each have an individual interpretation of what the clinical experience entails, there are also multiple layers and interactions that determine both a hidden and overt clinical curriculum. The core of the clinical curriculum contains three things: the authentic context of clinical or field work practice, the people involved in that context, and the process through which teaching and learning occur.

The clinical curriculum brings the practical realities of the health profession into juxtaposition with the academic curriculum. It emerges from practice and is situated in practice. The clinical context cannot be considered in isolation or manipulated or analysed apart from the social relationships that mediate it. Through the clinical curriculum, the processes that practitioners use to induct students into the discipline are acknowledged. As peripheral health professionals, students bring their academic culture to the authentic setting. Alongside accomplished practitioners, students respond to the realities of practice as they learn to become health professionals.

Practice for beginning health professionals is so imbued in the context that it is only in some precise clinical moments that teaching and learning can occur. So deeply contextual are these teaching and learning moments that the learning is in the experience and condition of the client and all that surrounds them. The opportunities and meaning-making for disciplinary knowledge development are facilitated and constructed through the immersion and discourse between the neophyte and experienced practitioners. Teachers in practice settings are acutely aware of assisting learners to develop hands-on technical skills and, while this is one goal, there are also others of equal importance. Interactions between the experienced practitioner, students, the client and those in the practice context help students to develop technical competence, interpersonal skills, professional standards of conduct, ethical and moral practices, and to become socialised into the profession. Thus the goals of clinical education are much broader, incorporating a number of key aspects of professional socialisation and practice such as:

- Application of classroom learning into 'real' contexts
- Socialisation into the chosen profession's standards and expectations
- Development of technical skills
- Development of professional attitudes, ethics and values
- Development of clinical decision-making processes
- Promotion of situation awareness for effective clinical decision making

- Promotion of cultural competence
- Experience working within the interprofessional team
- Development of understanding around the healthcare system
- Development of professional relationships and interactions with patients/clients, families and communities
- Development of an understanding of health within the broader social, cultural, political, economic and environmental contexts.

Clearly, the value of a positive clinical learning experience for any student cannot be understated. It has the potential to provoke passion for a particular practice area, prompt students to ask questions that may later transpose to a practice change or new research outcomes, and develop the profession further. Students' experiences in the clinical setting can directly influence their future career choices and, hence, the health workforce.

INSIGHT 1.1

Pause to consider your own teaching practice. Do you focus essentially on students' hands-on skills development?

In what ways do you, or could you, incorporate the achievement of broader education goals?

What experiences could you include to promote some of the other types of professional development?

Bridging Theory and Practice

Authors have argued for decades that a separation between academic and clinical practice exists, referring to the concept of a theory–practice gap. Similarly, others have contended its existence. However, the theory–practice gap may not be the result of differences between academic teaching and learning and experiences in clinical settings, rather the ability of the learner to transfer knowledge from one area to another. Situational factors such as the length of a course, a lack of familiarity with one's current clinical environment, short clinical placements, and differences between the pace of learning and that of clinical practice as contributing to impaired knowledge transfer may all have a role to play. Some clinical placements also take place within simulated settings, for example, as a result of no suitable placement being available, which adds further complexity. The practice partner plays a major role in assisting with the assimilation of classroom theory and clinical practice. In order to successfully achieve this, they need to have an understanding of the academic curriculum from which a student is emerging.

ACTIVITY 1.1

Understanding the curriculum background of a student will help reduce the existence of a divide between theory and practice. If you are a practice partner, prior to your next student clinical-placement rotation, source some information about their prior classroom learning. Ideally, obtain a copy of the course curriculum document. What theory has been covered to date?

How have clinical skills been taught?

What are the main concepts to be reinforced?

What are the practice expectations for the learner at the current stage of their curriculum?

Acquiring such knowledge can help to ensure seamlessness between the classroom and the practice environment. The establishment of a mutual partnership between the experienced practitioner and student highlights the need to reconcile the academic and practice worlds. Most experienced practitioners indicate they are aware that it is only through actual authentic practice that knowledge can be tested and extended (Billet & Henderson, 2011; Benner et al., 2011). These practitioners are aware it may be difficult for students to integrate the separate units of academic knowledge with the required synthesis of this knowledge in practice. Indeed it may be even more difficult for students to traverse two very different learning cultures. If a gap between academic and practical knowledge exists, experienced practitioners would appear well placed to try to bridge the cultural separation rather than perpetuate its divide.

CLINICAL COMPETENCE

One aim of clinical placements is to develop students' competence in their chosen fields. Many health professions have developed professional competency standards, required before one is licensed or permitted to practice in those professions. Hence, the achievement of required professional competencies or standards is often sought alongside set learning outcomes. Some examples are given in Table 1.1.

TABLE 1.1 Some Health Discipline Standards and Their Professional Bodies

Discipline	Professional Body	Standards
Nutrition and Dietetics	Dietitians Association of Australia	National Competency Standards for Entry-Level Dieticians
Midwifery	Nursing and Midwifery Board of Australia	National Competency Standards for the Midwife
Nursing	Nursing and Midwifery Board of Australia	National Competency Standards for the Registered Nurse National Competency Standards for the Enrolled Nurse
Occupational Therapy	Occupational Therapy Australia	Australian Minimum Competency Standards for Entry-Level Occupational Therapists
Pharmacy	Pharmaceutical Society of Australia	Professional Practice Standards
Physiotherapy	Australian Physiotherapy Council	Australian Standards for Physiotherapy

TEACHING ROLES FOR HEALTH PROFESSIONALS

Given that the goals of clinical education are broad in nature, the role of the practice partner is also diverse and complex. They are uniquely placed, intricately positioned between providing professional education and the site of care delivery. Fundamentally, clinical teachers need to be expert practitioners in their own right. Practice partners, however, could include practitioners at all levels of experience, including newly graduated professionals. Referring to the clinical teacher in medicine, but relevant across all of the health professions, Parsell and Bligh (2001) argue that 'Clinical teachers must possess a wide range of knowledge, skills and personal attributes and know when and how to apply them. In addition, knowledge of organisational and teaching strategies can help teachers to provide high quality patient care without eroding the quality of education' (p. 409).

A multitude of important clinical teaching role components have been described throughout the health professional literature, highlighting just how complex and multifaceted the role is. These components can be arranged into four key dimensions: professional practice, teaching and learning, management and support (Table 1.2).

TABLE 1.2 Dimensions of the Clinical Teaching Role

Professional Practice	Teaching and Learning	Management	Support
• Role model • Professional • Expert practitioner • Researcher • Client advocate • Coach	• Teacher/ instructor • Facilitator • Assessor • Questioner	• Supervisor • Negotiator • Communicator	• Career counsellor • Peer/critical friend • Student advocate • Resource person • Motivator

The components of the professional practice role include those surrounding the teacher's normal clinical role; that is, practising in a manner expected by the particular profession. The teaching and learning dimension follows the educational process and ensures learning outcomes. Management elements involve supervising student activity, and negotiating with health professionals for student experiences. Finally, the support dimension includes roles that provide for students' psychological wellbeing and additional aid in successful learning.

In many disciplines, such as medicine, clinicians directly provide clinical teaching for their students. While in others, there are specific roles to facilitate the delivery of clinical teaching. These are explored in more detail later in this chapter. Regardless of whether the role is a specific teaching one or not, effective clinical teaching in any of the health professions can be viewed as encompassing each of the above elements.

ACTIVITY 1.2

If you are currently working in a clinical teaching role, consider ways in which the role components listed above are incorporated into that role. Identify an example of when you undertake each role component.

If you are not working in such a role, observe or discuss with another clinical teacher their roles in day-to-day teaching. List examples of ways in which this person works across each of the identified role components.

CLINICAL TEACHING CONTEXTS

Clinical, or fieldwork, placements occur in a range of settings. Each setting offers unique opportunities for extending learning and enhancing the development of clinical skills.

Community Settings

These settings allow students to experience practice in environments where clients themselves exist. They allow students to understand how resource issues and social circumstances impact on the daily lives of clients and their families, or whole communities. They can occur in a vast array of settings, including the client's home, public or private clinics such as general practices or palliative care, or aged care facilities.

Acute Care Settings

These involve placement in settings where acute healthcare is delivered, primarily in hospital settings. These allow for understanding acute health needs and care delivery. For many health professional students, acute care settings allow for the development of a range of hands-on procedural skills to be developed.

Bedside Teaching

Occurring in acute care settings, bedside teaching is commonly described in medical literature but forms an important part of clinical education in other health professions, too. This teaching incorporates individual client factors into the educational process, using a real, case-based approach. It may involve a range of activities such as performing hands-on procedures or ward rounds.

Clinics both on and off Campus

These clinics are usually discipline-specific, specialised settings. In these instances, clients are often scheduled to meet with students and experienced practitioners.

Clinical Laboratories

These are usually recreated clinical settings within the university where students can safely practice clinical skills in a low-fidelity simulated context before entering clinical placements and performing these on clients. A number of disciplines such as medicine, nursing and physiotherapy use this approach to prepare their students for hands-on clinical skills development.

Clinical Skills and Simulation Centres

These are more specialised and higher-fidelity simulation settings. Learners enter contexts where they are able to practise their professional roles, often with other members of the healthcare team. They are often used to encourage high-level decision making and inter-professional teamwork.

Multiprofessional approaches to clinical learning, where different health professionals learn together, are becoming more common. Glen and Reeves (2004) assert that interprofessional education in nursing and medicine assists with developing professional identities and each profession's sense of belonging within the broader scope of healthcare provision. Interprofessional learning opportunities have been suggested as assisting in developing teamwork between different professional groups by providing increased awareness and recognition of one another's roles and breaking down professional 'silos'. The World Health Organization (2010) suggests that interprofessional education (IPE) is particularly beneficial for teaching:

- Teamwork
- Roles and responsibilities
- Communication
- Learning and critical reflection
- Relationships with, and recognising the needs of, clients
- Ethical practice.

DELIVERING EDUCATION

The Classroom

Within the academic setting, learning in the health professions involves a variety of classroom-based experiences. The primary ones are listed below:

- *Lectures* are the most common teaching approach and generally involve learning in large groups, which can sometimes number hundreds of learners. Lectures often deliver theoretical content that is built on through other learning experiences. One of the challenges with delivering lectures is meeting learners' needs and keeping them engaged and interested. Effective lecturers are those who can maintain learner engagement through the use of different teaching methods and interactivity.

- *Tutorials* involve small-group learning and consist of groups of up to 20 to 30 learners. These are more interactive and involve student activity in applying concepts learnt in lectures to practical situations. Effective tutorials facilitate individual learner responsibility and active engagement in learning. The tutor works to promote effective group functioning and allows students to work on problem solving.

- *Clinical laboratories*, or clinical skills centres, involve learners usually working in small groups in simulated clinical environments. They are designed to develop their hands-on (technical) and non-technical practice skills, such as teamwork and communication, to be applied later in 'real' practice situations. The teacher in this environment needs to possess sound clinical skills, the ability to work systematically with learners through skills learning, and provide constructive feedback that promotes ongoing development.

Online Learning

Increasingly in higher education, teaching and learning in the health professions is taking place through the use of emerging online media technologies such as Wiki©, blogs, YouTube and formal learning-management systems such as Moodle™ and Blackboard©, to name a few. Online learning offers new opportunities to make learning more flexible and accessible to learners who might not otherwise be able to access education. It also allows learners to tailor their learning time within their busy lifestyles. The teacher using online learning has a role in actively facilitating learner interaction and engagement through their online presence in order to allow desired learning outcomes to be achieved.

Clinical Placements

In clinical placements, students are exposed to their particular health profession environment in a health service or community setting. These facilitate professional socialisation and practice in the specific discipline. They should build directly on classroom learning experiences, allow for refinement of practice, and build exemplars and critical reflection for future on-campus and clinical learning. Clinical placements vary greatly in structure, not only between professions, but also within individual professions. For example, placements may:

- Be intermittent block placements from one week at a time to a full semester in length
- Be continuous placements of set days each week over the academic semester
- Consist of a few hours up to full 8-hour or 10-hour days
- Involve shift work, including nights and weekends
- Be supernumerary (unpaid) and, in a few circumstances, paid placements.

TEACHING RELATIONSHIPS AND MODELS

Many different models exist for the delivery of clinical teaching across the health professions. Some of these have specific titles, while others do not. A diversity of clinical teaching approaches within individual disciplines also exists, which further complicates this area. However, as highlighted in a review of different models used in physiotherapy, Lekkas et al. (2007) argue that no particular model for the delivery of clinical teaching is superior to another. Certainly, the nature of the individual clinical context will have some impact on the model most suitable for implementation there. The different models described in the literature can be classified into three groups: one-to-one clinical teaching, teacher and multiple students, and other models. Table 1.3 summarises those now described.

One-to-One Clinical Teaching

In these models, a student engages in a one-to-one relationship with a clinician who also assumes responsibility for both client care and student learning. A number of disciplines use the term 'preceptor' to refer to this model, including medicine, nursing, dentistry and pharmacy (Billay & Myrick, 2008). Flynn and Stack (2006) assert that the preceptor–student relationship falls in between teaching and mentoring. It is a relatively short relationship, usually only over the length of a particular clinical placement. It has set learning goals that need to be achieved rather than personal goals that characterise mentoring relationships.

A range of benefits and limitations of one-to-one (preceptor) models have been identified in health professional literature. The model offers the student the opportunity to have individualised attention (Lekkas et al., 2007; Yonge & Myrick 2007) rather than sharing the clinical teacher with other students.

Similarly, however, limitations to one-to-one models have also been reported. It has been suggested that these models require more time commitment than others (Lekkas et al., 2007). Acting in such roles has been widely reported as stressful for clinicians who also carry clinical workloads. Support and recognition for the role has been argued as important to ensure clinicians continue to be willing to adopt preceptor roles in the future (Hautala, Saylor & O'Leary-Kelley, 2007).

TABLE 1.3	Key Aspects of Different Common Health Professional Teaching Roles
Academic	An experienced health professional appointed within a university
	Academic roles may involve a combination of teaching and research, or be purely teaching focused or research focused
Clinical Teacher/ Facilitator	A recognised university-appointed representative with particular expertise, the Clinical Facilitator promotes academic knowledge as they supervise students' practical learning. The Clinical Facilitator operates from a formal educative role, straddling the university and practice arenas. Usually responsible for a number of learners
	No clinical workload
Clinical Teaching Associate (Secondee)	Individual seconded from a healthcare agency
	Usually no clinical workload when teaching
	Returns to usual clinical workload on completion of teaching secondment
Preceptor	A one-on-one teaching relationship
	Preceptor retains clinical workload
Mentor	Provides guidance on professional and personal development, but not usually direct clinical teaching
	Often a long-term relationship
Buddy	Student works alongside a clinician in providing client care. No clinical teaching expectations
	May be as short term as one day
Practice Partner	Similar to buddy, but an educative and socialisation relationship where the student is engaged in all professional activities alongside an experienced practitioner
	May be a short-term or long-term, one-on-one relationship
Peer Teacher	Student engaged in teaching another student. Teacher may be at the same level as the learner, or a senior student may engage in teaching a junior student

One Teacher with Multiple Students

In many health disciplines, one teacher assumes responsibility for the clinical education of a number of students. In nursing, this model was implemented following the transfer of education into the higher education sector. Here, one faculty member could be responsible for the full supervision of 8 to 12 students and does not carry a client load. While other models for the provision of clinical education have since been implemented, this model is still used in many areas. However, it is important to note that where one clinical teacher is responsible for a number of students, each may receive less clinical supervision than in one-to-one relationships. This model can be further complicated by the clinical teacher having to divide their clinical caseload equally across all students.

The Clinical Teaching Associate (or Secondee) was a subsequent variation on the model prompted by the need for clinical teachers with a greater familiarity with clinical environments. This particular approach has been reported in nursing literature since the late 1980s. Here, the clinical teacher, the Clinical Teaching Associate, is seconded away from their usual clinical practice role to support a group of students for the duration of their clinical placement. The position is remunerated by the university and, on completion of the placement, the teacher returns to their regular clinical practice role.

Other Models

Some other models have been introduced through the literature in the context of clinical teaching. However, while these may have informal components of clinical teaching, most are not technically clinical teaching models in themselves. Nevertheless, it is pertinent to recognise the roles they may have in the clinical environment.

Mentor

Mentoring is often used incorrectly interchangeably with preceptorship. Similarly, it involves the development of a one-to-one relationship. However, this role focuses on professional, personal and career development; in other words, the development of a mentee's career, both in the short and long term. A senior professional enters into a relationship with a junior person to provide professional guidance, not direct supervision or teaching.

Buddy

This construct emerges largely from within the nursing literature. Brammer (2006) describes this role as an informal relationship whereby a student works with a clinician. However, this is more of a caretaking role than an educational one. The role is responsible for client care delivery but does not incorporate any expectation of clinical teaching provision on the part of the clinician. The length of the relationship may be as short as one day.

Practice Partner

This is similar to the Buddy relationship but it is one that includes clinical teaching alongside direct client care. The practice partner model is an educative and socialisation model acknowledging that experienced practitioners have the knowledge and skill to help direct student learning while delivering care such as providing interventions or rehabilitation. A reciprocal relationship develops where students feel valued as a part of the professional community they are entering and confident to raise questions and assist in the practice of the profession. The experienced practitioner acknowledges their role as they facilitate and induct the student into becoming a safe, competent practitioner who will be a future colleague and representative of the health profession.

Peer Teaching

Peer teaching involves students teaching students. It may involve students at the same level of education or senior students teaching juniors. This approach has been increasingly described in a number of disciplines, including medicine, nursing, physiotherapy and occupational therapy. Peer teaching can be particularly beneficial for developing students' confidence and skills development and reinforcing the peer teacher's own knowledge.

INSIGHT 1.2

Reflect on the clinical teaching models used in your workplace. What factors have influenced the chosen approach?

Have other models been used? If so, what have been their benefits and limitations?

CHALLENGES IN CLASSROOM AND CLINICAL SETTINGS

Unlike teaching in a classroom, in clinical teaching there is a number of participants—including students, clients, their families and other health professionals—which adds to its complexity but also offers different opportunities. Furthermore, clinical teaching and learning often occurs within challenging environments over which teachers may have little control. Clinical teachers need to be cognisant of the effects of these environments and develop ways to promote optimum teaching and learning outcomes for students, regardless. It needs to be recognised that clinical teaching takes place in settings primarily designed for the management of healthcare so that client contact is central. Hence, the delivery of quality care is the key influence and desired outcome in those areas. Spencer (2003) notes that increasingly clients are choosing not to consent to student participation in their care. In this context, students may at times feel as though their learning needs are unimportant.

Client populations are transient and this can have a flow-on effect with regard to clinical teaching opportunities. Clients with conditions aligning to students' clinical learning needs for a particular placement may not be available and this requires some creativity on the part of the clinical teacher (Hoffman & Donaldson, 2004). Therefore, teaching can often be opportunistic. In addition, increasing client acuity and shorter inpatient stays can reduce the amount of direct involvement that students can play in a client's care.

Health professionals are increasingly reported to be stressed and overworked. The increased client throughput challenges opportunities for learning experiences. This is compounded by the growing demand for clinical places (Bennett, 2003) across many disciplines. Students may be seen as an additional burden or an extra pair of hands to help with care demands. In these situations, clinical teachers need to encourage clinicians to view students primarily as learners with learning needs, not as workers (Gaberson & Oermann, 2007).

As previously identified, in some settings, the clinician is also the clinical teacher. This requires responsibility for the provision of client care as well as student teaching. Available time and competing demands can complicate both roles, meaning that either one or both may receive inadequate attention. This can be further compounded in a context where there is little recognition paid to clinicians who also take on clinical teaching responsibilities (Spencer, 2003). Careful planning of the workload is needed in these situations to ensure both clients and students receive the necessary attention. Table 1.4 summarises these clinical setting challenges.

While one must be mindful of the challenges in clinical teaching, it is important to consider the overwhelming benefits that clinical experience in the 'real' setting offers students and their learning.

TABLE 1.4 Teaching and Learning Challenges in the Clinical Setting

• Focus on delivery of client care	• Staff workloads and stress
• Types of client conditions	• Uncontrollable, unpredictable environment
• High client acuity	• Competing demands
• Shorter inpatient stays	• Time constraints

Classroom environments expose students to standardised client-care situations where they can make basic links between theory and practice, develop beginning skills, and learn the benefits of problem-solving approaches to care. However, clinical practice offers opportunities to apply that learning further to 'real' clients with their own individual variations. They allow students to socialise into their chosen profession and develop a sense of their own professional role and identity. They allow students to engage in the interprofessional nature of health-developing capabilities available within the interprofessional team (Smith & Seeley, 2010). Table 1.5 summarises some clinical setting benefits.

INSIGHT 1.3

Reflect on the provision of clinical or fieldwork education in your own discipline area. What models are used to deliver this aspect of the curriculum?

Do these models have particular benefits and disadvantages?

Who are the key stakeholders in the practical teaching process?

What particular challenges are faced in the delivery of clinical education?

TABLE 1.5 Benefits of Learning in the Clinical Setting

• Exposure to 'real' clients	• Practice informs future learning and theory
• Professional socialisation	
• Development of professional identity	• Development of hands-on skills
• Application of classroom theory to practice	• Interprofessional engagement
	• Integration of work and learning

📷 SNAPSHOT

This chapter provides an overview of clinical teaching in the health professions. It explores the different roles undertaken by clinical teachers, and the contexts and structures in which clinical teaching occurs. It highlights some of the many challenges inherent in successful clinical teaching practice.

REFERENCES AND FURTHER READING

Benner, P., Stuphen, M., Leonard, V. & Day, L. (2010). *Educating nurses: A call for radical transformation*. San Francisco: Jossey-Bass.

Bennett, R. (2003). Clinical education: Perceived abilities/qualities of clinical educators and team supervision of students. *Physiotherapy*, 89(7): 432–440.

Billay, D. & Myrick, F. (2008). Preceptorship: An integrative review of the literature. *Nurse Education in Practice*, 8(4): 258–266.

Billet, S. & Henderson, A. (2011). *Developing learning professionals: Integrating experiences in university and practice settings*. Professional and practice-based learning series. Dordrecht, NLD: Springer.

Bluteau, P. & Jackson, A. (2009). *Interprofessional education: Making it happen*. London: Palgrave Macmillan.

Brammer, J. (2006). RN as gatekeeper: Student understanding of the RN buddy role in clinical practice experience. *Nurse Education Today*, 26(8): 697–704.

Flynn, J.P. & Stack, M.C. (2006). *The role of the preceptor: A guide for nurse educators, clinicians and managers* (2nd ed.). New York: Springer.

Gaberson, K.B. & Oermann, M.H. (2007). *Clinical teaching strategies in nursing* (2nd ed.). New York: Springer.

Gallagher, P., Carr, L., Wang, S.-H. & Fudakowski, Z. (2012). Simple truths from medical students: Perspectives on the quality of clinical learning environments. *Medical Teacher*, 34(5): e332–e337.

Glen, S. & Reeves, S. (2004). Developing interprofessional education in the pre-registration curricula: Mission impossible? *Nurse Education in Practice,* 4(1): 1–8.

Grossman, S.C. (2007). *Mentoring in nursing: A dynamic and collaborative process.* New York: Springer.

Hautala, K.T., Saylor, C.R. & O'Leary-Kelley, C. (2007). Nurses' perceptions of stress and support in the preceptor role. *Journal for Nurses in Staff Development,* 23(2): 64–70.

Hoffman, K.G. & Donaldson, J.F. (2004). Contextual tensions of the clinical environment and their influence on teaching and learning. *Medical Education,* 38(4): 448–454.

Lekkas, P., Larsen, T., Kumar, S., Grimmer, K., Nyland, L., Chipchase, L., Jull, G., Buttrum, P., Carr, L. & Finch, J. (2007). No model of clinical education for physiotherapy students is superior to another: A systematic review. *Australian Journal of Physiotherapy,* 53(1): 19–28.

McKenna, L. & French, J. (2011). A step ahead: Teaching undergraduate students to be peer teachers. *Nurse Education in Practice,* 11(2): 141–145.

Morison, S., Boohan, M., Jenkins, J. & Moutray, M. (2003). Facilitating undergraduate interprofessional learning in healthcare: Comparing classroom and clinical learning for nursing and medical students. *Learning in Health and Social Care,* 2(2): 92–104.

Parsell, G. & Bligh, J. (2001). Recent perspectives on clinical teaching. *Medical Education,* 35(4): 409–414.

Rodger, S., Thomas, Y., Dickson, D., McBryde, C., Broadbridge, J., Hawkins, R. & Edwards, A. (2007). Putting students to work: Valuing fieldwork placements as a mechanism for recruitment and shaping the future occupational therapy workforce. *Australian Occupational Therapy Journal,* 54(supp. 1): S94–S97.

Smith, P.M. & Seeley, J. (2010). A review of the evidence for the maximisation of clinical placement opportunities through interprofessional collaboration. *Journal of Interprofessional Care,* 24(6): 690–698.

Spencer, J. (2003). ABC of learning and teaching in medicine: Learning and teaching in the clinical environment. *British Medical Journal,* 326(7389): 591–594.

World Health Organization. (2010). *Framework for action on interprofessional education & collaborative practice.* Geneva: WHO.

Yonge, O.J. & Myrick, F. (2007). Preceptorship pathways for the senior undergraduate nursing student. In L.E. Young & B.L. Paterson (Eds), *Teaching nursing: Developing a student-centred learning environment.* Philadelphia: Lippincott Williams & Wilkins.

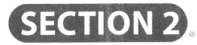

Foundations for Supporting Learning

CHAPTER 2.

Learners in the Health Professions

KEY CONCEPTS

- Types of learners in the health professions
  - Baby Boomers
  - Generation X learners
  - Generation Y learners
  - Culturally and linguistically diverse learners
  - Adult learners
- Theories underpinning teaching and learning
  - Adult learning theory
  - Experiential and social learning theories
  - Learning and cognitive styles
- Critical thinking and clinical reasoning
- Developing from novice to expert
- Learner expectations of the practice learning environment
- Stress in the clinical setting

INTRODUCTION

Students in the health professions are vital to the future of their disciplines and the delivery of healthcare. Effective education is fundamental to ensuring that health professionals are prepared for the future challenges in healthcare, not only those of the present. Profiles of learners in the health professions have changed markedly over recent years (Spuur et al., 2012). While many students are school leavers, an increasing number are entering via other studies, professions and occupations (McKenna & Vanderheide, 2012). In addition, more students are emerging from diverse cultural and linguistic backgrounds (Salamonson et al., 2012). The growing, resulting variety of students creates complexity and challenges for those involved in supporting their education, especially in the clinical practice setting.

This chapter introduces different types of learners commonly encountered in clinical education, some of their specific characteristics and the challenges in supporting their learning. It introduces theories underpinning clinical and workplace learning and suggests strategies for enhancing clinical learning opportunities and experiences. Finally, the chapter explores learners' common expectations of workplace learning environments.

WHAT WE KNOW ABOUT LEARNERS IN THE HEALTH PROFESSIONS

TYPES OF LEARNERS

Today's learners in higher education are more varied than in the past. Many health professional students are school leavers entering tertiary studies for the first time. However, there are increasingly more non-school leavers entering health disciplines, particularly with the growth of graduate-entry health professional programs. These people enter their studies with a raft of prior life experiences and learning and may be seeking a life change from work in another field. Their prior experience and perceptions can enhance the clinical learning experience but can also be challenging for those involved in facilitating their learning. In addition, these individuals may bring other challenges into their clinical experience, such as holding part-time employment to support their studies, and juggling family responsibilities with or without the support of a partner or family. Hence, their clinical placement experience may be just one of a number of priorities for the week.

The diversity of learners in health professions goes beyond school leavers and non-school leavers. Some learners may be re-entering their chosen profession after an extended time away. In addition, our multicultural society and policies to increase the enrolments of international students are leading to a greater number of culturally and linguistically diverse students being included. Each group of learners has its own particular challenges in clinical learning. However, while considering such facts as age and cultural background, it is important to remember each individual will have their own particular characteristics that will influence their clinical learning and performance. In this section, we will explore some of the characteristics of different learners in the health professions and identify challenges that they and their educators may face, along with ways to enhance the clinical learning experience. In the discussion to follow, we explore issues surrounding reported generational differences in learning, gender aspects and the issues for culturally and linguistically diverse learners.

Baby Boomers

The Baby Boomers include those people born between 1943 and 1960 (Zemke, 2001). They were educated in contexts where the teacher was the expert and provided the necessary information to learners based on what they considered to be important. Thus learning in this group was largely dependent on and guided by others.

Baby Boomer learners in the health professions are often seeking new employment opportunities and can bring with them years of learning and experience from a diversity of fields. In the educational setting, these students are often well prepared and punctual (Johnson & Romanello, 2005). Baby boomer learners are described as process driven, wanting 'to know the "what" and "how" before learning the "why" in a new situation' (Mangold, 2007, p. 21). Furthermore, this generation of learners may have undertaken the majority of their education without the use of computers. Yet, it is important to recognise that many will have embraced technology and possess advanced skills.

Generation X Learners

Generation X incorporates those individuals born between 1960 and 1980 (Zemke, 2001). This group has been reported to value its leisure time, with time being viewed as precious. They strive to have skills that are useable and seek both employment and financial security (Johnson & Romanello, 2005). Generation X learners need to be able to see the reason for doing something; that is, the value of their actions (Collins 2004). According to Johnson and Romanello (2005, p. 214), Generation X learners 'want things presented in a straight-forward manner and want to learn the information in the easiest and quickest way possible'. They can work in a self-directed, independent way but also enjoy working in teams (Billings & Kowalski, 2004; Collins, 2004).

Generation Y Learners

Generation Ys are known by many different titles such as 'Millenials', the 'Internet Generation', 'Nexters' and 'Generation Why'. They were born in or after 1982 to around the late 1990s, and have their own distinct learning styles. This generation have grown up with tech-nology all around them: computers, electronic games, mobile phones and so on. Hence they are technologically literate and can multitask well. The Internet and social media play a major role in their learning. While this generation can use technology, they may still require assistance to know how to find certain information to support their

learning. In addition, it is important to recognise that some Genera‑
tion Ys may have come from backgrounds that have limited their
exposure to technology.

In their learning, Generation Y learners reportedly enjoy working
in teams, so group activities work well. They also enjoy experiential
activities where they can test real-life experiences such as through
simulation and virtual reality (Billings & Kowalski, 2004). They are
self-confident and expect a highly structured learning environment
(Zemke, 2001), but they also expect immediate feedback on their
activities (Johnson & Romanello, 2005).

Regardless of demographic background, it is important to
recognise that each of the generational groups will encompass
different types of individuals with different learning approaches and
prior experience. White and Kiegaldie (2011) argue that all teaching
for all generational groups should include diversity and interactivity
to reflect individuality within each group. Thus it is important to
recognise individual differences and learning needs and styles within
any teaching activity.

ACTIVITY 2.1

Consider the different generations of learners you work with. How
appropriate do the descriptions described above fit those individuals'
approaches to learning in the classroom or clinic?

From your experience, how differently do the generations tackle their
learning requirements?

Are there particular challenges that present with each of the generations?

List what strategies you could put in place to facilitate optimal learning
for each of the different generations.

Culturally and Linguistically Diverse Learners

Culturally and linguistically diverse (CALD) learners may include international students, local students born overseas as well as students born locally. Hence, within the group there can be diversity of its own. Many of these learners can experience a number of particular challenges while undertaking their courses. Studies of nursing students from non-English-speaking backgrounds have identified a range of particular issues influencing their experiences (Salamonson et al., 2007; Tsukada & McKenna, 2004). In one study, Tsukada and McKenna (2004) found that international nurses studying nursing in Australia experienced struggles and challenges with:

- The English language and medical terminology
- Cultural differences that influenced making Australian friends and dealing with clinical practice experiences
- Different approaches to classroom learning and clinical learning environments
- Feelings of isolation and loneliness
- Financial difficulties.

It is important when working with culturally and linguistically diverse (CALD) students to take time at the commencement of the clinical rotation to understand any individual cultural and language issues that may impact on their learning. This enquiry may include exploring their experiences with learning and the nature of healthcare delivery in the country from where they originate. O'Connor (2006) suggests that CALD students can experience difficulties with applying concepts in the practice environment, and communicating with staff, clients and others. In the first instance, O'Connor recommends encouraging the use of concept maps and such support resources as bilingual dictionaries to assist with transition to the clinic.

However, effective communication is mandatory for practice across the health disciplines. If difficulties are not sufficiently addressed by these strategies, academic staff should assist with developing plans for overcoming difficulties. This should be done sooner rather than later, allowing time for the interventions to foster success in the clinical rotation (see Table 2.1).

TABLE 2.1 Promoting Learning with CALD Students

- Explore students' prior experiences of education and healthcare.
- Explore students' understanding of local cultural issues relating to their practice experience.
- Use concept maps to assist students to make sense of classroom learning in a clinical setting.
- Encourage students to participate in English conversation through interacting with other students.
- Encourage the use of support resources that may assist in understanding classroom and clinical learning experiences.

Adult Learners

All learners in the health professions are adults, whether school leavers or not. This brings with it numerous challenges that may infiltrate their learning experiences. Many of these learners are often financially supporting their own education, or supplementing other financial support. It is not unusual for learners in some disciplines to hold one, two or more paid employment roles throughout the duration of their courses. In addition to outside work, many have family and other commitments. They may have children or be caring for other family members. The time and effort required during clinical placements put further additional stress upon many students. Hence, supporting students in practice placements needs to be sensitive towards students' individual demands.

ACTIVITY 2.2

Consider the diversity of learners you regularly encounter in your teaching area.

(a) Discuss with colleagues:
   What potential challenges do learners face in that setting?
   What potential challenges do staff members hosting these learners face in clinical settings?

(b) Write a list of strategies which can support all of the stakeholders in promoting effective learning.

THEORIES UNDERPINNING TEACHING AND LEARNING

Learning in health professional courses is complex, involving a variety of learning environments. Clinical settings can be more complex than classroom learning environments. Learners are not only applying theory into the practice of their chosen field, they are socialising into the culture of the profession. This next section introduces some of the key theories that underpin learning and how these apply in the clinic.

Adult Learning Theory

Technically all learners in the health professions are adult learners, although some may not easily make the transition from school-based to higher education learning. Malcolm Knowles (1978) used the term 'andragogy' to describe adult learning, as opposed to 'pedagogy', which describes the ways children learn. Knowles described a number of characteristics that define adults in their approaches to learning, including:

- Adults have particular motivation driving their learning, such as obtaining a qualification or new career.
- Their learning is centred on what they need to know.
- Adults can be self-directed and take responsibility for their own learning.
- Adults have a readiness to learn things that apply to practice.
- Previous experience forms a basis on which subsequent learning can occur.
- Learning needs to be readily applicable to practice.
- Adults have the ability to problem solve.

Learning experiences, therefore, should be constructed in a way that recognises and respects what the learner brings to the situation. Table 2.2 suggests some approaches to facilitating effective learning for the adult learner.

TABLE 2.2 Enhancing Learning for Adult Learners

- Acknowledge the learner's previous learning and cultural experiences.
- Understand and build upon the entry knowledge and skill of each learner.
- Encourage the learner to be engaged in developing shared learning goals and outcomes.
- Include the learner in planning learning experiences.
- Allow the learner to explore areas of individual interest.
- Acknowledge outside influences that may place additional pressure on student learning.
- Foster mutual respect.

Experiential and Social Learning Theories

Learning in practice settings is significantly more complex than that which takes place in a traditional classroom. Not only are learners applying their classroom theory to real clinical practice, they are becoming part of a larger social world that is their chosen field. Furthermore, they are learning from the often-complex experiences taking place around them. Kolb (1984) describes the experiential learning cycle, a cyclical process by which people learn from their experiences. There are four phases in the cycle: the learner starts with concrete experience, moves on to a process of gathering observations and reflecting on the experience, and then develops abstract concepts and generalised ideas that are then tested in new situations. From here, the cycle repeats itself.

Bandura's social learning theory (also known as observational learning theory) provides yet another dimension to consider in relation to health science learners and the clinic. The foundation of Bandura's theory is that people learn by observing others, or role modelling. Given the importance of role modelling for learners in health professions, this approach is particularly relevant to clinical learning. Bandura describes four processes by which learning through role modelling occurs:

- *Attention*: Paying attention and observing the behaviour
- *Retention*: Remembering the characteristics of the behaviour
- *Motor reproduction*: Being able to carry out the behaviour
- *Motivational processes*: Recognising a need for the behaviour to be learned.

Role modelling is applicable to the development of practical skills. However, role modelling also plays a powerful part in teaching learners professional behaviours, attitudes and values. Poor role models in the practice setting have the potential to negatively impact on learners' development. By recognising and reinforcing positive role modelling, teachers can promote effective student learning and professional role development.

ACTIVITY 2.3

Consider the experiential and social learning theories discussed above and how these impact on student learning in your discipline.

Identify and list the types of professional characteristics that learners are expected to develop in your discipline.

Find two research articles that investigate how learners might experience and develop these characteristics in your teaching setting.

Reflect on and identify the key concepts in the articles. Add these reflections to your teaching portfolio.

. . . .

Learning and Cognitive Styles

Another factor that influences learning is that of cognitive or learning style; that is, the way in which people prefer to learn. Understanding learning styles can assist educators implement strategies to support student learning that suits their individual learning style. Kolb's (1985) learning styles inventory (LSI) is one of the most commonly reviewed. In this he describes four distinct types of learner:

- *Convergers*: These types of learners prefer to apply ideas to practical situations.
- *Divergers*: These learners prefer to explore concepts in order to generate new ideas.
- *Assimilators*: This group prefers to use logical reasoning and problem solving to develop new models.
- *Accommodators*: These have an adaptive approach; they enjoy new situations and environments, often taking trial-and-error approaches.

Honey and Mumford (1992) further developed Kolb's learning style inventory, varying the four learning styles. They describe the following types of learner:

- *Activists*: These learners concentrate on what is happening now. They need new experiences to continue learning.
- *Reflectors*: These like to observe cautiously before taking action themselves. They need to take time to review, research and consider.
- *Theorists*: These people take a logical, theoretical approach to learning, hence need purpose and structure. They may need time to explore ideas.
- *Pragmatists*: These learners like to test ideas, using problem solving to sort through learning. They like to apply their learning into real situations.

Another approach was taken by Neil Fleming (2006) who developed the VARK model. This approach identifies learners as:

- *Visual learners*, who learn best by seeing
- *Auditory learners*, who learn best by hearing
- *Kinaesthetic* or *tactile learners*, who learn best by doing.

Numerous studies have explored health professional learners and their preferred learning styles. Some of these are summarised in Table 2.3.

Table 2.3 also highlights some important aspects to be considered when engaging students in the health professions. While learning styles' research has some value for educators, some degree of caution is required. For this reason, learning styles work has received criticism.

TABLE 2.3 Reported Learning Styles in Health Professions

Authors	Discipline/s	Tool Source	Findings
Fowler (2002)	Radiography	Kolb (LSI)	Predominantly convergers or assimilators
French et al. (2007)	Occupational therapy	Kolb (LSI)	Tended to be divergers and convergers
Contessa et al. (2005)	Surgery	Kolb (LSI)	Primarily convergers
Rassool & Rawaf (2007)	Nursing	Honey & Mumford	Primarily reflectors
Zoghi et al. (2010)	Nutrition and dietetics, nursing, midwifery, occupational therapy, paramedics, pharmacy, radiation therapy, radiography, social work	Kolb (LSI)	Primarily convergers, with diverger and accommodator least preferred

As reflected in Table 2.3, similar groups can respond in different ways; that is, there is no one specific learning style for any professional group. Furthermore, it is important to consider that learners may regularly use different approaches to suit the particular learning tasks. Therefore, teaching needs to incorporate a range of approaches for learning outcomes to be optimal for all learners. Learning activities should be designed to extend individual learning needs for all learners. Teachers should also be aware of their own learning style preferences and consider how they influence their own teaching.

ACTIVITY 2.4

What implications do learning styles have for your teaching work?

How might you meet the needs of learners of all the different styles within your setting?

Use the Internet to source a learning styles questionnaire and examine your own learning style.

Consider what this says about you as a teacher. Write a reflection on how you can use the results to improve the way you teach and add to your teaching portfolio.

Promoting Clinical Reasoning

Many learners in the health professions are engaged in curricula underpinned by problem-based learning approaches. Such approaches seek to develop skills in learners that include problem solving and clinical reasoning, skills which are crucial to the development and delivery of high-level client care. Problem-based learning involves providing learners with a problem (usually through a scenario) that they need to solve. This requires learners to identify, individually or in small groups, what they do not understand, collect the resources that will assist in solving the problem, and work towards solving the problem. Issues and questions arising out of the problem are then discussed at the end of the process within the larger group. In the clinical setting, encouraging approaches that require learners to solve problems or issues can achieve a greater depth of learning and application of knowledge.

The use of questioning can also contribute to the development of sound critical thinking and clinical reasoning skills, and may greatly enhance the clinical learning experience. Questions are considered to be low or high level. Low-level questions may require a standard, factual response and little, if any, reasoning and consideration. High-level questions require the learner to think critically. Here the learner needs to apply learned knowledge to formulate a response, not just rely on memory. This approach is known as Socratic questioning and is 'systematic, disciplined, and deep, and usually focuses on foundational concepts, principles, theories, issues or problems' (Paul & Elder, 2007, p. 36). Learning Resource 4 provides information you may find helpful for developing questioning techniques.

ACTIVITY 2.5

Select a topic relevant to your practice area. Write a series of practically relevant questions you could ask learners related to this topic. Consider the potential for each of the questions to stimulate critical thinking. Are they low or high level?

How might you reformulate any low-level questions so that they encourage deeper thought?

••

DEVELOPING FROM NOVICE TO EXPERT

It is commonly voiced in clinical settings that staff are unclear of what stage individual groups of learners are at in their development and what they can and cannot do in practice. Clearly, learners undergo a developmental process from a position where they are able to perform minimal clinical procedures and spend a lot of time in observational roles, to gradually acquiring an increasing repertoire of skills they can perform. However, some learners will also be better prepared for certain clinical areas than others. For example, a student may be in their final year but rotated into a specialised field for which they have not been fully prepared. In addition, individual students will get to 'master' skills at different rates.

Patricia Benner (1984) describes the journey from novice to expert in nursing students, having applied a model previously developed by Dreyfus and Dreyfus (1980). The key aspects of her model are broadly applicable into other health disciplines and may assist educators to understand learners' levels of preparedness for practice in certain clinical areas. Benner describes five developmental stages through which nurses progress:

- *Novice*: This person is completely new to the situation where they will practice. In the case of health professionals, they have learned classroom theory but not applied this to practice.

- *Advanced Beginner*: This person 'can demonstrate margin-ally acceptable performance' (Benner, 1984, p. 22). They have experienced sufficient realistic situations to be able to recognise important aspects.
- *Competent*: This person has developed the ability to plan care and has refined clinical skills. According to Benner, while this person is able to cope with many situations, they may not yet be able to practise with speed and flexibility. It is at this level that the majority of graduates will exit their university courses.
- *Proficient*: The proficient practitioner has enhanced percep-tion. They have learnt from significant experience and can plan appropriate care in response.
- *Expert*: Finally, the expert practitioner has acquired immense knowledge and experience, can perform high-level clinical decision making and can manage very complex situations. This level may take many years to reach, if at all.

These levels are not necessarily permanent. In a new setting, an individual may revert back to lower levels because they do not possess the knowledge and experiences of that particular area. The majority of learners will fall into the novice and advanced beginner categories. Often they spend short, concentrated periods of time in any clinical area and then may move to a completely new one. By the end of their courses, though, it is anticipated they have reached a competent level.

ACTIVITY 2.6

Examine the learners in your teaching setting. At what level/s would you consider they are practising? Compare your analysis with the expecta-tions of clinical staff of learners' performances. Are the clinical staff members' expectations realistic? Discuss with your colleagues.

At what levels might clinical staff be practising? How do they self-determine at what levels they might be practising? How could you use this information to support learners? Record your findings to inform your future teaching practice.

STUDENT EXPECTATIONS OF THE PRACTICE LEARNING ENVIRONMENT

Learners often enter clinical practice with different expectations than staff may hold. Learners are motivated by their own learning requirements and needs. However, practice environments exist for the purpose of delivering healthcare to clients. This can at times result in tensions and challenges that may become the practice partner's responsibility to resolve. This requires an understanding of the different perspectives and working towards negotiating a resolution suitable to both parties.

Research has been conducted to explore the characteristics of clinical learning environments. Papp, Markanen and von Bonsdorff (2003) explored Finnish nurses' perceptions of their clinical environments. These authors found that learners saw a 'good' clinical environment as one where there was positive co-operation between staff, where learners were regarded as colleagues, appreciated, included as part of the team, and where staff were positive about mentoring them. Positive environments had a sound philosophy underpinning care, and care was delivered at a high standard. Finally, there was co-operation between the school and clinical staff.

STRESS IN THE CLINICAL SETTING

Clinical placements can be extremely stress-provoking for learners. Learners are entering settings that are often unpredictable, dynamic and uncontrollable. They may be unfamiliar with the healthcare agency, its policies and procedures, the staff and client mix, and enter as outsiders who may be in the setting for only a short time. Learners commonly fear not knowing what might be expected of them, performing procedures on 'real' clients for the first time, or not feeling welcome in the clinical setting.

Medical students have been found to experience stress relating to feelings of inadequacy in providing client care and feeling they have

Insufficient knowledge (Radcliffe & Lester, 2003). Similarly, nursing students have reported stress when performing skills for the first time and questioned their own lack of experience (Shipton, 2002).

Despite this, most learners have the ability to adapt well to new learning situations. The teacher in the clinical setting plays a significant role in supporting learners to recognise aspects that may impact such anxieties and stresses, and enabling learners to manage them. In addition, the teacher is a lynchpin in assisting learners to identify the contribution they can realistically and confidently make to the individual clinical setting (see Table 2.4).

TABLE 2.4 Strategies for Enhancing the Clinical Learning Environment

- Explore with learners their fears and anxieties, seeking to effectively manage them.
- Provide clinical staff with information about the learners and their learning needs prior to commencement of the placement.
- Encourage staff to include learners as valued team members.
- Provide extensive orientation materials for learners to familiarise themselves with the setting.
- Ensure staff mentoring or precepting learners are those who will be positive role models for learners to emulate.
- Choose learning experiences where staff morale and quality of care is high.
- Explore with students their initial expectations of the placement and, where possible, facilitate access to learning opportunities.
- Work with learners to identify learning objectives specific to the clinical setting.
- Promote ongoing communication lines between the university and clinical site throughout the placement experience.
- Provide opportunities throughout the placement to evaluate learners' experiences and facilitate two-way feedback.
- Guide learners in identifying the unique contribution they can make to the clinical setting.
- Nurture and value learners as future care providers in their discipline.

ACTIVITY 2.7

Consider your own practice setting. Imagine coming into that environment as an outsider. What particular aspects may enhance learning experiences?

Identify what features may provoke anxieties.

Develop a range of strategies you could develop to ease the learners' transition into the area.

📷 SNAPSHOT

This chapter explores the nature of learners in the health professions. It highlights the increasing diversity and complexity that this stimulates in classroom and clinical settings, and how particular characteristics can influence the learning process. The chapter also introduces a number of theoretical considerations for clinical learning and looks at ways in which the practice partner can optimise learning experiences.

REFERENCES AND FURTHER READING

Benner, P. (1984). *From novice to expert.* Menlo Park, California: Addison-Wesley.

Collins, D.E. (2004). Workplace diversity: A generational view. *Radiologic Technology,* 76(1): 62–68.

Contessa, J., Ciardiello, K.A. & Perlman, S. (2005). Surgery resident learning styles and academic achievement. *Current Surgery,* 62(3): 344–347.

Dreyfus, S.E. & Dreyfus, H.K. (1980). A five-stage model of the mental activities involved in directed skill acquisition. Unpublished report supported by the Air Force Office of Scientific Research, USAF, University of California Berkeley.

Fleming N.D. (2006). *Teaching and learning styles: VARK strategies*. Christchurch, New Zealand: N.D. Fleming.

Fowler, P. (2002). Learning styles of radiographers. *Radiography*, 8: 3–11.

French, G., Cosgriff, T. & Brown, T. (2007). Learning style preferences of Australian occupational therapy students. *Australian Occupational Therapy Journal*, 54(1): S58–S65.

Honey, P. & Mumford, A. (1992). *The manual of learning styles* (3rd ed.). London: Peter Honey.

Johnson, S.A. & Romanello, M.L. (2005). Generational diversity: Teaching and learning approaches. *Nurse Educator*, 30(5): 212–216.

Jones-Devitt, S. & Smith, S. (2007). *Critical thinking in health and social care*. Los Angeles, CA: SAGE.

Knowles, M. (1978). *The adult learner* (2nd ed.). Houston: Gulf Publishing.

Kolb, D.A. (1984). *Experiential learning: Experience as the source of learning and development*. Englewood Cliffs, NJ: Prentice Hall.

Kolb, D.A. (1985). *The learning style inventory* (rev. ed.). Boston, MA: McBer and Co.

Mangold, K. (2007). Educating a new generation: Teaching baby boomer faculty about millennial students. *Nurse Educator*, 32(1): 21–23.

McKenna, L. & Vanderheid, R. (2012). Graduate entry to practice in nursing: Exploring demographic characteristics of commencing students. *Australian Journal of Advanced Nursing* (online), 29(3): 49–55.

Montana, P.J. & Lenaghan, J.A. (1999). What motivates and matters most to generations X and Y. *Journal of Career Planning and Employment*, 59(4): 27–30.

O'Connor, A. (2006). *Clinical instruction and evaluation* (2nd ed.). Boston, MA: Jones and Bartlett.

Papp, I., Markkanen, M. & von Bonsdorff, M. (2003). Clinical learning environment: Student nurses' perceptions concerning clinical learning experiences. *Nurse Education Today*, 23(4): 262–268.

Paul, R. & Elder, L. (2007). Critical thinking: The art of Socratic questioning. *Journal of Developmental Education*, 31(1): 36–37.

Radcliffe, C. & Lester, H. (2003). Perceived stress during undergraduate medical training: A qualitative study. *Medical Education*, 37(1): 32–38.

Salamonson, Y., Everett, B., Andrew, S., Koch, J. & Davidson, P.M. (2007). Differences in universal diverse orientation among nursing students in Australia. *Nursing Outlook*, 55(6): 296–302.

Salamonson, Y., Ramjan, L., Lombardo, L., Lanser, L., Fernandez, R. & Griffiths, R. (2012). Diversity and demographic heterogeneity of Australian nursing students: A closer look. *International Nursing Review*, 59(1): 59–65.

Shipton, S.P. (2002). The process of seeking stress-care: Coping as experienced by senior baccalaureate nursing students in response to appraised clinical stress. *Journal of Nursing Education*, 41(6): 243–256.

Spuur, K., Caroline, L., Falconi, C., Cynthia, M., Cowling, C., Bowman, A. & Maroney, M. (2012). Demographics of new undergraduate medical imaging and medical sonography degree students at CQUniversity, Australia. *Radiography*, 18(2): 117–122.

Tsukada, T. & McKenna, L. (2005). Factors influencing international nurses when studying nursing in Australia. *Asian Journal of Nursing Studies*, 8(1): 32–40.

White, G. & Kiegaldie, D. (2011). Gen Y learners: Just how concerned should we be? *The Clinical Teacher*, 8(4): 263–266.

Zemke, R. (2001). Here come the Millenials. *Training*, 38(7): 44–49.

Zoghi, M., Brown, T., Williams, B., Roller, L., Jaberzadeh, S., Palermo, C., McKenna, L., Wright, C., Baird, M., Schneider-Kolsky, M., Hewitt, L., Sim, J. & Holt, T.-A. (2010). Learning styles preferences of Australian health science students. *Journal of Allied Health*, 39(2): 95–103.

CHAPTER 3

Situating Learning and Learning Communities

KEY CONCEPTS

- Situated learning
- Workplace learning and legitimate peripheral participation
- Professional socialisation
- Socio-political influences on clinical learning
  - Nature of clinical settings
  - Constraints on clinical teaching
  - Interprofessional considerations

INTRODUCTION

As we explored in the previous chapter, learning is a complex undertaking. The number of factors that influence learning as well as relational theories can quite easily overwhelm the teacher and make it difficult to decide how to assist the learner. An added layer to how we teach is that we teach in an often multifaceted workplace. Unlike other workplaces, the clinical area is a learning triad of teacher, learner and client. Clinical or fieldwork learning for health professionals acknowledges that different curricula operate in workplaces, be they explicit or tacit, as health professionals undertake the work of the profession and manage client conditions.

This chapter presents a theoretical perspective to better understand workplace learning. The conceptual background lets us view the workplace and the interactions within it as a rich, contextual learning environment. As learners enter the workplace, their learning through working alongside accomplished practitioners becomes both an occupational and professional necessity.

SITUATED LEARNING: WHAT THE LITERATURE REVEALS

This section examines the available literature to provide an educative structure with which to aid an understanding of how we interpret clinical experiences. The historical account provides an educative platform that has been used by present researchers (Billet & Henderson, 2011) to provide explanations of contextual learning that takes place between the experienced practitioner and the learner entering professional practice.

In early discussions on workplace learning, Dewey (1933) subscribed to the belief that education should take place within a community rather than in isolation from the community. He recommended there should be a close relationship between the academic and workplace environments to assist cognitive development and action.

Much later it was proposed that, in order for people to live and grow, their individual cognitive and psychological development needed to be understood in their own system of social relations or community (Vygotsky, 1978). This view of cognitive socialisation focused more on collaborative cognitive activity as a source of development rather than intrinsic individual cognitive activities that were developed by others such as Piaget (1971).

Vygotsky (1978) suggested that individual intellectual development is embedded in a social and cultural environment that fosters conceptual growth through tools for thinking and partners who are skilled in the use of such tools. (Other aspects of this development will be explored in Chapter 6.) Vygotsky was convinced that the primary 'tool' allowing this to occur was internalisation of culture and history through the ways in which society and culture influenced the development of language and discourse within a community (Wertsch, 1986). We can see this as we examine how each individual health professional has developed and continues to use unique language as the principal source to exchange knowledge.

INSIGHT 3.1

Consider the historical roots of your profession. Think about the symbols, customs and shared meanings that are part of your professional culture.

Now, examine the language and jargon you use in your everyday communications with your professional co-workers.

How does this influence your learning environment and how you induct learners and newcomers into your professional community?

Often we are unaware of the profound affect that just being surrounded by experienced practitioners can have on learners. Exchanges, both verbal and non-verbal, with experienced practitioners in the clinical environment, 'embody a culture's intellectual history; they have theories built into them, and users accept these theories—albeit unknowingly—when they use these tools' (Resnick,

1991, p. 7). It is this tacit knowledge that has stored the personal and collective history of a culture, a social history, of the health professional that is carried into each act of interaction and from one generation to the next. This helps us to explain how the experienced practitioner builds up exemplars and theories of practice over time and uses these to inform new situations incorporating elements of familiar features from previous experiences.

However, we can ask ourselves, how do we go about helping the learner interpret, understand and develop these communal cognitive tools? In an effort to understand how shared meaning is created, Vygotsky (1978) coined the term 'zone of proximal development' to describe the characteristics of learning as behavioural change. Vygotsky subscribed that changes in behaviour occurred through shifts in control and responsibility and defined the zone of proximal development as:

> … the distance between the actual developmental level as determined by independent problem solving and the level of potential development as determined through problem solving under adult guidance or in collaboration with a more capable peer. (Vygotsky, 1978, p. 86)

Given the opportunity to carry out joint cognitive processes that are more advanced than learners could manage independently, joint problem solving with an experienced practitioner has the potential to serve as a basis for subsequent independent activity. In essence, this recognises the significant contribution that joint problem solving and collaborative reflection with more experienced practitioners can have on the development of becoming a health practitioner. However, Vygotsky also developed a theoretical framework that merged social institutions, culture, activities and cognition. He referred to this work as a theory of activity (Davydov & Radzikhovski, 1985).

Briefly, this theory is seen to occur when individuals are involved in the practical activities (the structure of labour) that incorporate the psychological tools (cognitive processes) of a particular culture

(Bruner, 1985); in this case, healthcare professionals. Bruner offers support to Vygotsky's view on learning:

> ... there is a deep parallel in all forms of knowledge acquisition—precisely the existence of a crucial match between *support system* in the social environment and an *acquisition process* in the learner. I think it is this match that makes possible the transmission of the culture. First in a set of connecting ways of acting, perceiving, and talking, and finally as a generative system of taking conscious thought, using the instruments of reflection that the culture 'stores' as theories, scenarios, plots, prototypes, maxims, and so on. (Bruner, 1985, p. 28; italics in original text)

Vygotsky maintained that individuals need to make conscious associations with past experiences for learning to become functional and incorporated into the mind for use in future situations. The result of Dewey, Vygotsky and Schon's (1933; 1978; 1983) theorising is that, for learning to be meaningful, it needs to be located within the practice or the culture of the practice. To this end, cognitive psychologists began exploring teaching and learning within these communities of practice. They referred to this as 'situated cognition' (Collins, Brown & Newman, 1989; Damarin, 1994; Damon, 1991; Lave, 1988; Resnick, Levine & Teasley, 1991; Wertsch, 1986).

These researchers argued that 'the social context in which cognitive activity takes place is an integral part of activity, not just the surrounding context for it' (Resnick, 1991, p. 4). Damon (1991) identified three explanations that have come to be associated with situated cognition. He viewed them as firstly denoting:

> ... practice-centered knowledge, as distinct from knowledge that is abstract, decontextualised and rule-bound. Second, the term has been used to suggest a scientific approach that views thinking as a form of action rather than merely as disembodied and solipsistic reflection. Third, the term has been used to assert that all cognition is embedded in

historical, cultural and social-relational contexts. In this socio-cultural application, cognition is seen to be spawned by social interaction and communication. In use it is seen to be widely distributed across individuals and collectives. (Damon, 1991, pp. 384–385)

Here we can clearly see that the underlying premise of situated cognition and thus learning (sometimes referred to as situated learning, situated knowledge or socially shared cognition) is the placement of the learner in real-life contexts rather than the often abstract academic environment. Indeed, this assumption has continued as tertiary learners now spend considerably more time than previously in different workplaces to experience client interactions and professional practice 'first hand'.

WORKPLACE LEARNING AND LEGITIMATE PERIPHERAL PARTICIPATION

Legitimate peripheral participation (LPP) is a process where a learner or 'newcomer' to the discipline moves towards becoming a full-participant 'old timer' or from an advanced beginner to expert in a community of practice. In this book, they are learners involved in the community of healthcare practice. Legitimate peripheral participation is a process through which learners initially participate on the periphery of a socio-cultural community of practice. Over time they move towards centripetal participation, becoming more engaged and more active within any discipline's overall practices (Lave & Wenger, 1991).

By virtue of their learning status, the learner cannot be involved as a full participant in all aspects of activities of the practice. Thus, participation is from the periphery. At the same time they are not passive observers but must be recognised as being legitimate members of the community. Under the guidance of an experienced practitioner, newcomers develop mastery of knowledge and skills of the community of practice as they move towards full participation in the socio-cultural practices of that community. Participation indicates interaction, not just with the activities of the community of practice but with all those experienced in the community of practice. A community of practice can be defined as a group of professionals, in this case health professionals, with particular skill or expertise who have a shared enterprise and interact formally in an organisation, in a networked way, to achieve shared pragmatic and knowledge-related goals (Hakkarainen et al., 2004).

The transition of the learner to graduate entering the heart of the profession can only be understood through their relations with experienced practitioners in their community of practice. It is by being immersed in the community of practice that the heritage, culture, knowledge, skills and attitudes of the profession can be appreciated and learned. It is the relationship between the learner as a newcomer and the experienced practitioner who holds and translates the socio-cultural knowledge that facilitates this process.

INSIGHT 3.2

A criticism of Lave and Wenger's work by Fuller et al. (2005) is that it needs to be acknowledged that there are different degrees of peripherality for the learner/novice compared with the experienced worker entering a different field of the same profession.

As a mechanism of enculturation, for a learner, LPP also includes relationships, not just between learners and experienced practitioners, but other participants, skills, the artefacts, symbols and ideas that are part of the culture of the practice. Participation further involves technologies or tools of the trade. This is especially significant because the artefacts—such as hands for touching, a stethoscope, spirometer, blood pressure monitor, goniometer, doppler or ultrasound machine—operate within a cultural practice that carries a substantial proportion of that profession's practices and heritage.

ACTIVITY 3.1

What professional tools do you use? Which ones are used by other health professionals?

How does your use of these tools differ from other health professionals' use of the same artefact?

How do you think this information is used to maintain the cultural practices of your profession?

Do the tools, artefacts and symbols of your practice perpetuate or constrain your profession?

How do they influence the culture of your professional practice?

Involve the learner and a number of your colleagues in this discussion.

Inherently, learning to use the 'tools' of the profession is a way to connect with the history of the practice and to participate more directly in its culture (Lave & Wenger, 1991). Learning as a characteristic of social interaction cannot be extricated from its legitimate context. As such LPP is not a pure instructional method; rather, it is an orientation for observing and understanding learning in new ways in the workplace.

Schon's (1987, p. 36) work supports this stance indicating that:

> … when someone learns a practice, he (sic) is initiated into the traditions of a community of practitioners and the practice world they inhabit. He learns their conventions, constraints, languages, and appreciative systems, their repertoire of exemplars, systematic knowledge, and pattern of knowing in action. (Schon, 1987, p. 36)

It is senior practitioners who initiate learners into the traditions of practice. The traditions of practice are viewed as 'the customs, methods and working standards', and 'initiation into the tradition is the means by which the powers of learners are released and directed' (Dewey, 1933, p. 151). Correspondingly, learners cannot be told what they have to know but discover, with guidance, the ways of knowing in and of the profession.

Through the relations within a practice, learners learn how to share in the community. The shared practices create an environment that includes both 'talking within' to share information about ongoing activities, and 'talking about' the practices and activities through stories that support 'communal forms of memory and reflection' (Lave & Wenger, 1991, p. 109).

As the novice and more experienced practitioner share information and reflect, they both reproduce and transform the community of practice. Both bring their own unique individual characteristics, biographies and trajectories of learning and practices of the profession to the relationship and activities of the community. As the learner/newcomer becomes involved in the practice guided by the experienced practitioner, both their knowledge and the community of practice inevitably change. The transmission, reproduction and transformation of professional knowledge are therefore dependent and embedded in this co-participation (Evans et al., 2006).

Legitimate peripheral participation relies on involvement with experienced practitioners. Access to the community of practice—that is, access to a range of ongoing activities, experienced practitioners, resources and opportunities—is the key to LPP. Access provides learners with the opportunity to engage in the culture of the workplace as they are immersed in the practice (Billet & Henderson, 2011). Through legitimate peripherality the learner is provided with unique opportunities to make the culture of practice theirs, gradually assembling a general idea of what constitutes the profession. According to Lave and Wenger:

> This might include: who is involved; what they do; what everyday life is like; how masters talk, walk, work, and generally conduct their lives; how people who are not part of the community of practice interact with it; what other learners are doing and what learners need to learn to become full practitioners. It includes an increasing understanding of

how, when, and about what old-timers collaborate, collude, and collide and what they enjoy, dislike, respect and admire. It offers exemplars (which are grounds and motivation for learning), including masters, finished products in the process of becoming full participants. (Lave & Wenger, 1991, p. 93)

Throughout LPP an assumption has been made (Lave & Wenger, 1991) that the experienced practitioner is at liberty, and has the skills and willingness, to be involved with the learning of the newcomer/ novice. This is not always the case. Indeed, it has been identified that three other important dimensions can impact on the relationship: that experienced practitioners are willing to have their knowledge questioned; that at some point the newcomer will replace the experienced practitioner; and that it is through the experienced practitioner that the learner gains access to learning resources, including the client (Lave, 1993).

ACTIVITY 3.2

Consider how you and your fellow experienced practitioners react to the above three important dimensions. Discuss how you might minimise their impact on learners entering your practice area.
••

No matter what model is used, or how you work with learners, the role of the experienced practitioner will assist the learner in the cultural ways of knowing, particularly in an authentic context through reflection and guardianship. Lave (1988) and Lave and Wenger (1991) propose that through the support of an accomplished practitioner, learners gain access to cultural knowledge and practices of the community, in order to understand their symbolic relationships with the people in the practice and to develop an identity as a member of the profession. To its credit, LPP draws attention to key aspects of learning experiences located in workplaces, and the practice of a profession, that may be overlooked in traditional educational frameworks.

Learners build a progressive identity of themselves as they co-participate in the authentic context or the 'lived in world' of where practice occurs in the midst of experienced practitioners. Learners are producers of learning, not work. However, learners use the work within the specific discipline context to inform their learning. Through their encounters with the workplace, learners experience, transform and internalise their interpretations of practice. Even as they hover on the periphery of the practice realities, they create meaning out of the practice. Legitimate peripheral participation acknowledges that, for the learner, 'being in' the professional context with an accomplished practitioner does indeed facilitate the transformation of knowledge and construction of identity as a health professional.

PROFESSIONAL SOCIALISATION

Moving from the theoretical positions on workplace and situated learning, it is timely then to explore the nature of professional socialisation into the health professions. Ajjawi and Higgs (2008) define professional socialisation as:

> … being both an individual's journey of professional development and a social, acculturation process occurring within a professional group and context, [it] provides a dynamic frame of reference for learning to reason, both at university and in the workplace. (Ajjawi & Higgs, 2008, p. 133)

Professional socialisation includes learning the foundational skills and knowledge necessary for the specific profession, as well as the development of reasoning and decision-making skills required of the professional (Ajjawi & Higgs, 2008). This can be a particularly complex area for clinical teachers and new students to deal with as initial perceptions collide with practice realities. Richardson et al. (2002) explored new physiotherapy students' views of that profession. They found that students entered their courses with different ideas on the roles of physiotherapists and these were informed by a range of influences, including careers teachers, friends and the media. In nursing, Howkins and Ewens (1999) found that students had their own ideas about the profession based on their personal experiences. While little is known about other health professions, it is likely that the situation is similar. Therefore, in assisting students to socialise into their chosen professions, educators play a role in challenging students' entry beliefs and attitudes.

The development of students' professional identities emerges through their clinical placement experiences and working alongside professionals who are assisting their adaptation to the environment and the healthcare team. Secrest et al. (2003) explored the meaning of professionalism for baccalaureate nursing students. Students in their study described feeling the need to belong in clinical settings, and this included being valued within nursing teams. They also valued having knowledge and being competent in practice as well as receiving affirmation from others to build their sense of being a professional. Interestingly, the development of profession-specific social networks has been attributed to professional socialisation (West et al., 1999). Hence, professional socialisation plays a powerful social and professional role in an individual's development.

ACTIVITY 3.3

Reflect on your own profession and how new students are socialised into it. What are some of the challenges they experience?

Determine the strategies you could employ to minimise any difficulties that students confront.

SOCIO-POLITICAL INFLUENCES ON CLINICAL LEARNING

A range of challenging social and political influences can impact on the delivery of clinical teaching and learning. As explored in Chapter 1, it should be remembered that, while we are teaching the next generation of health practitioners, we do so in organisations whose primary purpose is to treat and respond to a range of clients and their conditions, not principally to promote learning. Hence the needs of clients will take precedence over students' learning needs. As a teacher it is important to be cognisant of the tensions this can create for students who may have learning needs that need to be covered in a short space of time, while also ensuring clients' needs are promptly addressed.

Nature of Clinical Settings

The nature of the clinical learning environment is unlike that of the classroom setting. According to Papp et al. (2003) it is diverse and influenced by many factors, including the physical ward settings and health professionals, teachers, clients and their families. These authors argue that, while the academic setting is controlled, the clinical learning environment is impossible to control. This challenges the teacher in fostering learning and developing the rapport to facilitate access to practice experiences.

Over the course of their studies, many students will also rotate through a variety of clinical sites. Each one has its own ways of doing things, its own distinct culture which, for students, can be difficult to enter and navigate. Each environment has social relationships between staff members who are well established and have acknowledged or unacknowledged understandings. A student can easily feel like an intruder or isolated. Such feelings are not conducive to effective learning. Hence, students quickly have to develop an understanding of the social climate in the setting and their place within that culture. In their study, Papp et al. (2003) found that nursing students valued feeling appreciated in clinical practice when they were included as part of the team. Similarly, in a study with medical students, Dornan et al. (2005) concluded that students' uncertainty in the clinical setting could diminish their motivation, while social interaction improved motivation. For effective learning to commence, the teacher in the practice setting thus has an important role in facilitating a student's entry into the social network within the individual setting.

ACTIVITY 3.4

Consider your own clinical practice area. What social and professional networks exist there?

How easy is it for transient learners to become included in those networks?

If barriers exist, explain how you might ease students' transition into the setting.

The dynamic nature of the setting poses further complications for facilitating learning. Clinical learning depends on access to clients. Learning objectives usually include the performance of procedures relevant to the particular health profession. However, one cannot predict the types of clients that will present at any time and what their particular needs might be. Hence, access to suitable learning opportunities may be problematic at certain times. Again, tensions can arise when students are unable to meet prescribed learning outcomes because suitable opportunities do not arrive. This may require the clinical teacher to be creative in assisting the learner to find alternative ways to meet learning requirements.

Constraints on Clinical Education

A range of factors may act to constrain the delivery of clinical education. These can provide challenges for practice-based teachers. In their work on clinical education in nursing, McKenna and Wellard (2004) identified a number of aspects emerging through the literature, including:

- The presence of increasingly acutely ill clients in general wards, making ward staff busier, less able to support students and understand their particular learning needs
- Students having less direct supervision and being exposed to more hazardous situations
- Sessional or casual nature of clinical teacher employment, making recruitment and retention difficult

- Fewer permanent and full-time staff available within clinical settings, resulting in the same staff having to work with students on a continual basis and leading to staff burnout.

Another issue increasingly faced by teachers is accessing appropriate clients to allow students to fulfil their learning requirements. It is not unusual to find a number of different health professional students in a particular practice setting, each with their own individual learning needs. Repeated student access to particular clients can result in the clients becoming overburdened by numerous requests for students to undertake different assessments and procedures on them. This may result in ward staff taking a 'gate keeping' approach to reduce the exposure of clients to some students. The situation presents a dilemma for the teacher who needs to explore other opportunities for students to meet their learning requirements.

ACTIVITY 3.5

Consider your own clinical setting. What factors promote effective clinical teaching?

What factors act to constrain teaching?

Identify ways to address some of the limitations.

Interprofessional Considerations

An individual client's care provision does not usually rely on just one type of healthcare professional. The nature of healthcare is such that it involves a number of different health professionals working together to achieve optimal care outcomes. Many universities provide curricula opportunities to promote interprofessional education (IPE) for their students, to enhance their professional teamwork, understanding and communication. Underpinning this approach is a perception that, if students learn together early in their professional preparation, they will work more effectively together later as qualified health professionals (Zarezadeh, Pearson & Dickinson, 2009). This then has the potential to enhance client care outcomes. Hence, teaching approaches that integrate learners from different professions have become increasingly popular over recent years.

There are many ways in which students from different disciplines can learn together. They may learn to develop professional attributes (such as empathy or communication) together, or work on client-based scenarios (or real cases) that require the specific knowledge of their own disciplines but which also promote working as a team. Interprofessional education activities encourage learners to examine their roles in client care, as well as those of other health professionals engaged in care delivery (Zarezadeh et al., 2009). Recent research suggests that generally students from various health professions are positive about this type of learning and value the promotion of teamwork (Williams et al., 2012).

Often, such interprofessional learning takes place in a simulation setting, where students take on their professional roles in a supported, simulated learning environment, responding to changing client circumstances. While research around such activities is currently limited, it has been suggested that interprofessional simulation-based education (IPSE) promotes student confidence, teamwork and communication (Gough et al., 2012).

ACTIVITY 3.6

Consider your own clinical teaching context. Are students from different professions encouraged to learn together? If not, list some ideas of how you might facilitate interprofessional learning activities.

📷 SNAPSHOT

Learners' interactions within practice settings play a vital role in their learning and professional socialisation. This chapter introduces a range of theoretical positions on workplace learning, which are aimed at providing an understanding of the development of health professional students. The powerful nature of professional socialisation is examined in light of these theories. This has been further extended into exploring the nature of clinical settings; how these settings have an influence on clinical teaching and learning. The discussion highlights the complex role of clinical teachers in facilitating students' access to appropriate clinical learning opportunities. In the following chapter, these aspects are further explored in the context of preparing for student learning in practice settings.

REFERENCES AND FURTHER READING

Ajjawi, R. & Higgs, J. (2008). Learning to reason: A journey of professional socialisation. *Advances in Health Sciences Education*, 13(2): 133–150.

Barr, H. & Low, H. (2012). *Interprofessional education in pre-registration courses: A CAIPE guide for commissioners and regulators of education*. London: CAIPE.

Billet, S. & Henderson, A. (2011). *Developing learning professionals: Integrating experiences in university and practice settings*. Professional and practice-based learning series. Dordrecht: Springer.

Bluteau, P. & Jackson, A. (2009). *Interprofessional education: Making it happen*. London: Palgrave McMillan.

Bruner, J.S. (1985). Vygotsky: A historical perspective. In J.V. Wertsch (Ed.), *Culture, communication and cognition: Vygotskian perspectives* (pp. 1–30). Cambridge: Cambridge University Press.

Collins, A., Brown, J.S. & Newman, S.E. (1989). Cognitive apprenticeship: Teaching the crafts of reading, writing and mathematics. In L.B. Resnick (Ed.), *Knowing, learning and instruction: Essays in honour of Robert Glaser* (pp. 453–494). Hillsdale, NJ: Lawrence Erlbaum Associates.

Damarin, S. (1994). The emancipatory potential of situated learning. *Educational Technology*, 34(8), 16–22.

Damon, W. (1991). Problems of direction in socially shared cognition. In L.B. Resnick, J.M. Levine & S.D. Teasley (Eds), *Perspectives on socially shared cognition* (pp. 384–397). Washington, DC: American Psychological Association.

Davydov, V.V. & Radzikhovski, L.A. (1985). Vygotsky's theory and the activity-orientated approach to psychology. In J.V. Wertsch (Ed.), *Culture, communication and cognition: Vygotskian perspectives* (pp. 31–58). Cambridge: Cambridge University Press.

Dewey, J. (1933). *How we think* (rev. ed.). Boston, MA: D.C. Heath.

Dornan, T., Hadfield, J., Brown, M., Boshuizen, H. & Scherpbier, A. (2005). How can medical students learn in a self-directed way in the clinical environment? Design-based research. *Medical Education*, 39(4): 356–364.

Evans, K., Hodkinson, P., Rainbird, H. & Unwin, L. (2006). *Improving workplace learning*. London: Routledge.

Fuller, A., Hodkinson, H., Hodkinson, P. & Unwin, L. (2005). Learning as peripheral participation of practice: A reassessment of key concepts in workplace learning. *British Educational Research Journal*, 31(1): 49–68.

Gough, S., Hellaby, M., Jones, N. & MacKinnon, R. (2012). A review of undergraduate interprofessional simulation-based education (IPSE). *Collegian*, 19(3): 153–170.

Hakkarainen, K., Palonen, T., Paavola, A. & Lethinen, A. (2004). *Communities of networked expertise: Professional and educational perspectives*. Amsterdam: Elsevier.

Hoffman, K.G. & Donaldson, J.F. (2004). Contextual tensions of the clinical environment and their influence on teaching and learning. *Medical Education*, 38(4): 448–454.

Howkins, E.J. & Ewens, A. (1999). How students experience professional socialisation. *International Journal of Nursing Studies*, 35(1): 41–49.

Lave, J. (1988). *Cognition in practice: Mind, mathematics and culture in everyday life*. Cambridge: Cambridge University Press.

Lave, J. (1993). Situating learning in communities of practice. In L.B. Resnick, J.M. Levine & S.C. Teasley (Eds), *Perspectives on socially shared cognition* (reprinted ed., pp. 17–36). Washington, DC: American Psychological Association.

Lave, J. (1997). The culture of acquisition and the practice of understanding. In D. Kirschner & J. Whitson (Eds), *Situated cognition: Social, semiotic and psychological perspectives* (pp. 17–35). Mahwah, NJ: Lawrence Erlbaum Associates.

Lave, J. & Wenger, E. (1991). *Situated learning: Legitimate peripheral participation*. Cambridge: Cambridge University Press.

McKenna, L. & Wellard, S. (2004). Discursive influences on clinical teaching in Australian undergraduate nursing programs. *Nurse Education Today*, 24(3): 229–235.

Papp, I., Markkanen, M. & von Bonsdorff, M. (2003). Clinical learning environment as a learning environment: Student nurses' perceptions concerning clinical learning experiences. *Nurse Education Today*, 23(4): 262–268.

Piaget, J. (1971). *Psychology and epistemology*. New York: Grossman.

Resnick, L.B. (1991). Shared cognition: Thinking as social practice. In L.B. Resnick, J.M. Levine & S.C. Teasley (Eds), *Perspectives on socially shared cognition* (pp. 1–24). Washington, DC: American Psychological Association.

Resnick, L.B., Levine, J.M. & Teasley, S.D. (Eds). (1991). *Perspectives on socially shared cognition*. Washington, DC: American Psychological Association.

Richardson, B., Lindquist, I., Engardt, M. & Aitman, C. (2002). Professional socialization: Students' expectations of being a physiotherapist. *Medical Teacher*, 24(6): 622–627.

Schon, D.A. (1983). *The reflective practitioner: How professionals think in action*. New York: Basic Books.

Schon, D.A. (1987). *Educating the reflective practitioner*. San Francisco: Jossey-Bass.

Secrest, J.A., Norwood, B.R. & Keatley, V.M. (2003). 'I was actually a nurse': The meaning of professionalism for baccalaureate nursing students. *Journal of Nursing Education*, 42(2): 77–82.

Vygotsky, L.S. (1978). *Mind in society: The development of higher psychological processes.* Cambridge: Harvard University Press.

Wertsch, J.V. (Ed.) (1986). *Culture, communication and cognition: Vygotskian perspectives.* Cambridge: Cambridge University Press.

West, E., Barron, D.N., Dowsett, J. & Newton, J.N. (1999). Hierarchies and cliques in the social networks of health care professionals: Implications for the design of dissemination strategies. *Social Science & Medicine,* 48(5): 633–646.

Williams, B., McCook, F., Brown, T., Palermo, C., McKenna, L., Boyle, M., Scholes, R., French, J. & McCall, L. (2012). Are health professional students 'ready' for interprofessional learning? A cross-sectional attitudinal study. *Internet Journal of Allied Health Sciences and Practice,* 10(3), available online at http://ijahsp.nova.edu/articles/Vol10Num3/williams.htm.

Zarezadeh, Y., Pearson, P. & Dickinson, C. (2009). A model for using reflection to enhance interprofessional education. *International Journal of Education,* 1(1): E12.

Creating Optimal Learning Environments

CHAPTER 4

Preparation for Learning

KEY CONCEPTS

- Preparing the environment for learners
  - Academic environment: Lesson planning, formulating learning outcomes
  - Clinical environment: Auditing clinical/workplace settings
  - Self-preparation
  - Briefing
  - Establishing relationships
  - Orientation and welcome
- Learner-centred preparation: Clinical contracts and portfolios
  - Negotiated learning agreements (learning contracts)
  - Learning portfolio development

INTRODUCTION

Preparation for learning assists the learner to consider their learning and basic requirements of the educational experience. For you, the teacher, it is an opportunity to prepare yourself, your material and the environment for the learner. Sound preparation is fundamental for optimising any learning experience.

Health professional learning begins during on-campus classroom teaching experiences and includes lectures, tutorials, workshops, laboratory, simulations, or blended learning. Such learning events incorporate the development and exploration of professional knowledge and skills within controlled and safe learning environments. Learners normally undertake skill development practice through a variety of low- and high-fidelity simulations, role playing and demonstrations, in conjunction with academics and practising professionals. In some cases, actors or consumers are employed to ensure realism and authenticity in the learning experience.

In both academic and clinical environments, learners are guided to use their knowledge to develop habits that assist their metacognitive learning; that is, learning about *how* they learn. This aids the transformation of learning across these two intrinsically linked environments.

In order to assist the learner, it is important you are familiar with the learner's broader university curriculum. Universities and professional courses espouse different philosophical approaches to teaching and learning as well as expectations of learner outcomes. Familiarising yourself with the learner's curriculum and the intent of practice experiences will demonstrate your commitment to preparing the next generation of health professionals, the environment and yourself, to plan and recognise beneficial learning and teaching moments.

As a new teacher, you may be designing both on-campus and off-campus learning events for learners. This chapter suggests preparatory approaches requiring input from both teachers and learners.

LEARNING ENVIRONMENT PREPARATION

PREPARING THE ACADEMIC ENVIRONMENT

The academic curriculum sets the overall scene for learning through the use of specific global objectives. Constructing learning requires careful alignment between the objectives of the curriculum, the course (sometimes also called the *program*), the unit of study, the individual class and clinical objectives. As you unpack the course objectives, you become able to develop meaningful and achievable segments of learning to be delivered, in a prescribed timeframe. Each class taught produces its own unique set of objectives and design possibilities.

Developing Learning Outcomes

Learning outcomes (or objectives) are statements that convey learner expectations and assist the teacher to structure learning events. Each begins with a verb and provides a set of instructions so the student can relate to the intent of the class and content to be presented, as well as what is expected of them. The way you plan to teach helps students not only to achieve the outcomes, it facilitates the rehearsal of how to learn and the future application and integration of the concepts taught.

To extend learning and the retention of content, assessment and grading should be directly related to the objectives. Formative and summative assessment (discussed in Chapter 7) reinforces for the student and teacher whether or not learning has occurred and outcomes have been achieved.

To assist the teacher to develop learning outcomes, Anderson and Krathwohl (2001) re-orientated Bloom and Krathwohl's (1956) original *Taxonomy of learning objectives*. This is an excellent resource for any teacher because they help construct learning outcomes. Primarily, well-developed learning outcomes:

- Are clear statements that can be measured
- Begin with a verb that indicates what the learner should be able to do with their knowledge or skills and at what level
- Are preceded by a stem that provides a timeframe for the learner
- Specify any conditions relating to level of performance
- Need to be achievable.

Examples of Learning Outcomes

On completion of this session, and with further practice, the learner should be able to:

1. Identify key members of the health professional team.
2. Discuss the importance of teamwork in client care delivery.
3. Demonstrate a beginning ability to work with other health professionals in the delivery of client care.

Here the above initial statement (or stem) identifies that the learning outcomes will require time beyond that in the classroom to achieve. The verbs used in each of the outcome statements all require a different level of application and performance. Learning Resource 2: Thinking Skills Framework provides a table of very useful verbs. The condition of 'a beginning ability' demonstrates the level at which the learner should be able to perform in practice. Many clinically oriented learning outcomes will require such conditions as this.

Establishing the learning objectives facilitates your ideas on how you will design the learning experience. These lead into the development of a lesson plan that provides a structure to assist in the preparation, delivery and management of the actual teaching session.

ACTIVITY 4.1

Identify a topic related to your teaching practice. Develop a set of achievable and measurable learning objectives for the topic. The following question sets offer suggestions.

Lesson Planning

First of all, begin your planning by asking: What is the aim of the session? This is what you, as the teacher, intend the teaching session to achieve.

Continue with identifying what type of class is to be delivered. Is it a lecture, tutorial, simulation, workshop, blended learning, web-based activities, online or self-directed learning?

What is the topic? Do you have the required knowledge?

Who are the learners? For example:

- Are they novice or experienced learners?
- What prior knowledge do they bring?
- What types of learners are they (see Chapter 2)?

Do you need to prepare the learner prior to the class: are there any previous activities they must undertake such as reading an article or book chapter, or undertaking a web-based learning activity?

What prerequisites (or assumed prior knowledge) are required to scaffold learning for this class?

What teaching resources are needed and available? Do you have access to them?

Where will the session be held?

How long is the session programmed to be?

What type of preparation will the learning environment require; for example, seating arrangements?

What are you going to do to actively engage the learners, for example:

- Gain and maintain their attention?
- Motivate them?
- Sequence the learning (moving from what is known to incorporate new or reinforced information)?

Learning Outcomes

Define the learning outcomes. For example: 'At the end of the class, students will be able to …'

How will you know the learner has achieved this? For example: 'Successful learning will be demonstrated by …'

What aids or barriers may have an impact on teaching and learning?

In answering these questions, you will also consider how you will go about teaching the class. This is a time when the teacher draws further on theories of learning and teaching to develop and use creative resources to support delivery. Breaking down the class content into smaller learning segments will assist your time management, ensuring all the learning outcomes will be achieved. Keep in mind it is easy to be distracted, so perform continuous self-checks to make sure you are not deviating from your plan. It is useful to keep your written plan beside you during the delivery of your session. While there is more than one approach, Learning Resource 3: Lesson Plans provides an example of how a lesson plan can be constructed.

Consider how comfortable you feel delivering the content. Rehearsing the session before the day can be very beneficial. Some presenters do this by standing in front of a mirror to see how they appear to an audience. Others video-record their rehearsal to review their performance.

On the day, ensure that the physical and social environment is conducive to learning. Check the climate—the temperature of the room—and the social climate such as seating arrangements. Try to minimise any potential distractions. This is particularly important if the teaching will occur in a clinical setting. Know how to use equipment and that it is operational. Have all your resources ready. Consider, too, there are certain times of the day that can impact on concentration and learning effectiveness, such as immediately after eating lunch, when you may need to work harder to keep learners engaged.

Delivery and Development

Some suggestions to help with delivery and development are:

- Let the learners know the intent of the presentation and how it links with previous and future sessions.

- Use variety to keep students interested. Some ideas are to present a short video and have students identify its key concepts. Present a client presentation or problem. Ask students to identify what it is they need to know and how they will go about finding and interpreting the information to make clinical decisions. Use their ideas to structure key concepts, initiate discussion, and generate dilemmas and debate.

- Prepare a range of questions as prompts for yourself to use through the class.

- Use references to support the content, demonstrating to students the use of evidence-based practices. Including hyperlinks to resources will aid your credibility and demonstrate to the learner how to think about and use resources.

- Use examples from practice. Draw on clients', learners' and your own experiences.

- Develop a range of strategies to deal with disruptive behaviours, including discussions that wander off on unrelated tangents.

- Use your voice and presence; for example, ensure you can be heard and check you are not using repetitive words that can be distracting for the learner such as 'All right', 'OK' and 'Um'. Do not remain still in one place or with one group of learners; move about to ensure all learners feel involved.

- Sequence learning segments. End by reviewing key aspects before moving onto a new concept. Better still, have students identify key points throughout the lesson and recapitulate and reflect on their learning at the end of the lesson. Learners can also share these ideas with one another in class or online.

- Develop different ways to reinforce student responses to your questions and/or redirect answers to build on concepts or topics under discussion.

- Vary strategies for students to think about and action links with newly generated knowledge and transformative practices.

- Conclude the class by summarising and revisiting the objectives, and linking the session with subsequent learning experiences.

INSIGHT 4.1

Take the time to reflect and identify aspects of your class that went well or you will change. Did you become aware of any particular personal mannerisms?

Evaluate how you will incorporate these reflections in your next class.

ACTIVITY 4.2

Using the template in Learning Resource 3, or another type, develop a lesson plan for the session for which you previously developed your learning outcomes.

PREPARING THE CLINICAL ENVIRONMENT

In most instances, the goals of the formal clinical experience are expressed as intended learning outcomes and stem from the academic curriculum. They can be content and professional-skill-development orientated; specific or broad. Knowing the platform on which you and the learner will engage is essential to a successful experience.

The context in which the learner is entering also requires analysis. Consider for a moment much of what you take for granted as you go about your day-to-day activities. These are: the environment (sight, sounds, smells); people (roles, relations, reactions, relationships); climate (social, political, economic); the learner's role in the practical setting (reflector, participant, observer, facilitator); and the personal and physical resources the learner may require to achieve practice goals in your area of work.

ACTIVITY 4.3

Reflect on and then document elements of the environment, people, climate and the learner's role. Learning Resource 8: Learning Environment Evaluation assists the teacher with assessing the effectiveness and suitability of the environment.

Think about what a learner would notice or need to know as they entered your work environment for the first time.

As the learner enters the often unfamiliar clinical environment, they look towards the clinical facilitator or practice buddy for direction and assistance to interpret the curriculum. Your job is to assist the learner to incorporate and adapt the academic curriculum to the clinical environment in which you work. Through your guidance, you help the learner to construct and construe knowledge and its relevance to their clinical experience.

Self-Preparation

Before you can begin to assist the learner, preparing yourself is necessary. As a practitioner you may be new to teaching and thus you are also a learner. As a reflective teacher, it is important you are aware of your strengths and limitations as a teacher and practitioner.

INSIGHT 4.2

What do I need to know about myself to become an effective and efficient teacher?

Consider where your ideas about teaching have originated. What made a good or bad teacher or experience for you?

Now identify what you consider to be your strengths as a teacher. Identify what you think your limitations are. Make a list of the ways you can develop your skills as a teacher.

Once you have a clear picture of yourself as a teacher you will be better able to assist others. Understanding who you are—your beliefs, idiosyncrasies, content and skill-level proficiency, strengths and limitations—provides you with the insight to develop continually and respond appropriately to change situations. From a clinical perspective, McAllister (2005) believes that teachers who are self-aware have a strong sense of finding meaning in their work, of accepting responsibility for student learning and client care while also seeing clinical education as a life-long endeavour.

BRIEFING

Following self-preparation, the second stage is the briefing session. Some health professionals refer to this as the pre-clinical conference. It can take place on campus and is recommended to occur on the first day of the placement in the practice environment. On campus, students may be given an overview of the academic faculty's expectations of the forthcoming experience. Students may also be requested to produce a range of information to prepare prior to entering the clinical environment. In Australia, current immunisation records and police checks are such examples. Furthermore, students may be asked to collect and integrate information for an upcoming assessment item, such as a theoretical paper, case study presentation, best-practice evidence or discussion presentation material related to their clinical experience.

In the clinical learning environment, briefing usually takes place at the start of the initial placement and, for some health professionals, on a daily basis prior to clinical encounters (Papaspyros et al., 2010). The initial placement briefing provides the foundation for all forthcoming experiences. MacKenzie (2002) defines briefing as an activity that orientates a learner to the experience. Briefing helps establish relationships and expectations while setting the scene and parameters of the experience. It includes instructions and rules required by the learner to successfully navigate, operate and achieve personal learning goals in the healthcare environment.

The unfamiliar and new experiences presented to learners in healthcare environments may be exciting as well as fearful. A briefing provides a quarantined period of time, set aside, for an individual or a group to anticipate and discuss, with the teacher, their thoughts and feelings and the potential learning opportunities and demands of the clinical or field experience ahead (Stockhausen, 1994). It is also an ideal time to ensure the learner feels safe and that processes are in place to create a safe learning environment.

To develop confidence, a briefing period can be scheduled prior to the learner undertaking an encounter with a client. This allows the learner an opportunity to rehearse and imagine what they will do, how they intend to do it and anticipate potential reactions (Benner et al., 2010). It can also be a time to extend the learner's appreciation of the client's circumstances, inclusive of socio-political and cultural factors. What works with a client in one situation may not necessarily work with another client in a different context. However, rehearsal has the potential to help prepare the learner to anticipate differences or similarities.

BUILDING RELATIONSHIPS

The briefing stage assists the teacher and learner to establish their relationship and the parameters and expectations of the practice experience. The initial meeting between the teacher and learner is sometimes awkward. Learners are frequently anxious because they are entering the often-unpredictable professional arena. Some learners lack confidence; others are overconfident and some are apprehensive about dealing with clients, their presentations and interacting with other health professionals. On the other hand, teacher-practitioners are busy. Often clinical areas are understaffed and the constant procession of learners in the environment can strain even the best clinical learning environments (Billet & Henderson, 2011).

However, as a place of learning and teaching for future health professionals, each party has particular expectations of the other. As the teacher you may expect a learner to show enthusiasm and be well prepared for the clinical experience. The learner may expect staff to be welcoming and accommodating and to have ready access to them when they need it. It is when these expectations are incongruent that the foundation for a professional relationship is displaced. It is essential then that, in a very brief period of time, an open, respectful and trusting learner–teacher or learner–practitioner relationship is established. The following processes can often help to establish rapport and create ease for the learner and teacher to communicate their feelings, thoughts, knowledge and experience.

ACTIVITY 4.4

Develop Understandings

Try to conduct the initial welcome away from interruptions. Both you and the learner need to demonstrate to each other and alert colleagues that the orientation and briefing is an important prelude to the overall experience.

Think about and then write down your expectations of the learner entering your clinical area, for example: What is my role and how will I assist the learner to learn?

Solicit from the learner their expectations of you as a teacher during the clinical rotation. Have them write these down. Ask them what they perceive your roles and functions are, for example: Let me know how you would like me to work with you, and what support you think you require.

Using the two lists, sit together and compare and discuss your expectations of each other. Consider where your lists deviate or converge and ways you can align your expectations. As the teacher, this is also an excellent time to ask yourself such questions as: Do I need to adjust my behaviour to meet the student's expectations? Are the student's expectations realistic? What behaviours do I bring to this relationship? Do I need to modify my expectations of the student to ensure success in the relationship?

Active listening, attending and encouraging remarks will ensure that each other's opinions are appreciated. Attending—through such positive non-verbal signals as maintaining eye contact, body leaning and being in a non-distractive environment—generates positive regard. Encouraging remarks such as, 'That's interesting' or 'Tell me more' promote involvement.

Once you have had the opportunity to discuss your expectations, develop several predetermined ground rules that identify ways for teaching and learning to occur. For example, confirm an understanding that:

- The boundaries of each other's roles are respected and client care is not compromised

- Treatment regimes are maintained

- 'Time Out' discussions are organised if either party requires a role clarification or feels there is a conflict that needs to be resolved

- There are pre-arranged signs, words or gestures that tactfully indicate you will intervene in client care. This avoids unnecessary interruption to care or embarrassment to the client or learner

- Time is allocated and structured during the day for negotiated learning and teaching episodes.

Negotiating and establishing such strategies ensures there are no miscommunications between both parties, that each one is fulfilling their role, and the relationship is maturing.

Ice Breakers

To break the ice with learners, teachers could ask such questions as:

- Tell me about the type of clinical experiences or field work you have already had?
- What subjects have you been studying this session?
- What areas of practice interest you most?
- What type of clients do you enjoy working with?
- What challenges you most in the clinical environment?

Think about other questions you could ask to help establish your relationship.

••

When you are establishing a collaborative, welcoming and well-distributed learning environment, always address the following aspects:

- Remember and use names
- Readiness: assess students' readiness to learn and your readiness for the learners
- Create a low-risk, non-judgemental atmosphere
- Reassure the learner they are not alone
- Set boundaries: understand the expectations of one another
- Generate interest by harnessing enthusiasm
- Gain insights
- Show mutual respect.

Research clearly indicates that learners who feel welcomed into the clinical environment will flourish (Billet & Hendersen, 2011). Easing learner anxieties and assisting the learner to work on the periphery and make the gradual transition into becoming a fully fledged member of the health profession hinges on a well-prepared orientation that includes the learner's expectations and opportunities to enhance and maximise their learning potential.

DESIGNING AN ORIENTATION PROGRAM

Because healthcare takes place in a variety of settings, there is no one orientation checklist that can be developed and used for general purposes. However, there are some common aspects that can be identified and adapted to clinical settings, as considered below.

INSIGHT 4.3

A well-prepared orientation helps the learner familiarise themselves to the setting. Investigate if your organisation already provides an orientation package. Evaluate if the package is comprehensive enough for the new employee or learner entering your clinical area. Keep in mind that the orientation will be slightly different for either the new employee or learner.

The new employee may require a more comprehensive orientation, whereas the learner may only be a short-term visitor and require enough orientation to function in the organisation safely and legally. Remember the orientation may be paper-based or online, with weblinks to guide the orientation and/or a self-guided tour. Here is a list of suggested information to include:

- A welcome statement
- The organisation's statements of purpose: vision, mission statement, aim, strategic plan, values
- Organisational structure: key personnel, services
- Specific information about the designated work area (e.g. diabetic podiatry clinic, private physiotherapy practice, intensive care unit, rehabilitation or residential aged care facility)
- Relevant organisational policies and procedures such as:
  1. Human resources
  2. Workplace health and safety

3. Emergency procedures

4. Infection monitoring and management

5. Clinical waste

6. Incident reporting

7. Documentation

- Key discipline-specific roles and responsibilities
- A map identifying key areas of importance
- Car parking or public transport services
- Staff amenities (meals and snacks, change areas, lockers, toilets)
- Library facilities
- Email and Internet/Intranet access
- Access details (e.g. swipe cards for secure areas).

Does your specific work area have its own orientation program? If so, evaluate it for its completeness. Add to it if necessary.

If your work area does not have an orientation, develop one.

Preparing Other Staff for the Learner's Experience

Remember it is not just you who will be assisting the learner but your whole work unit. It is courteous to announce to your colleagues the learner's expected arrival and any knowledge you have of the learner's anticipated experiences or expectations. Discussing and planning as a group how you can assist the learner to feel welcome and achieve their academic and personal goals will demonstrate to the learner that the clinical environment they are entering is willing to accept and assist them to become part of the profession. After all, the newcomer may eventually be a future work colleague!

ACTIVITY 4.5

Identify various ways you can welcome and invite students to be part of the workplace and team. You may also like to seek the workplace's expectations of you and the learner. These exercises help with building relationships, dispelling misinterpretations and clarifying others' roles and responsibilities in the workplace.

....

Preparing Clients for Students

Before involving clients in student's learning episodes, it is ethical to seek permission and consent from the person. Provide the person with information regarding their involvement and answer any question they may have. Allow time for the person to consider their involvement (Janicik & Fletcher, 2003). Once approval has been given, introduce the student—or the student may introduce themselves to the person—and identify what they will be doing and for how long.

ACTIVITY 4.6

How do you go about recruiting and preparing a client for student encounters?

....

LEARNER-CENTRED PREPARATION: CLINICAL CONTRACTS AND PORTFOLIOS

NEGOTIATED LEARNING AGREEMENTS (LEARNING CONTRACTS)

A negotiated learning agreement or learning contract is a document that maps a learner's plan to navigate their desired learning outcomes and processes in the practice setting. The contract is self-initiated; it gives the learner permission to explore areas of interest and control over their learning as they identify and utilise resources in the field to implement their strategies to demonstrate and evidence learning that fosters and leads to retention. Throughout this process, learners become self-directed knowledge scavengers, identifying and consuming facets of the field experience that leads to a transformative outcome.

Both the teacher and learners can benefit through the use of the learning contract (Kennedy-Jones 2005). The advantage to learners of instigating their own personal clinical objectives is that it forces the learner to reflect on and document what they are to consider: what they need to know to achieve a successful outcome, how they will demonstrate this, and how to evaluate if their learning has occurred. Engagement in this activity highlights to the learner their learning needs, generates interest and creates motivation to learn. There is a greater sense of ownership and commitment to the learning experience, leading to achievement. Staff benefit because they are alerted to areas of interest and required learning by the learners and they can then begin to negotiate mutually planned learning activities with the learner. As the teacher and experienced practitioner, you have built up a collective knowledge of the clients, staff and the organisation. With this knowledge you can support the learner-specific learning intentions. While supporting the learner in their endeavours, you can also broaden the learner's horizons, alerting them to nuances in the field, extending their learning, and exploring theoretical, evidence-based practice and novel ways to examine and respond to clinical events.

The learning contract can be initiated during the first briefing session, with refinements following discussion with you. The student may not yet have any idea of the type of clients they will be dealing with on a daily basis. Allowing the learner some time to assess and investigate clients and the environment will assist them to determine their learning requirements. Permitting learners to identify other resources, such as specific client needs or specialist departments within the clinical environment, will also enhance learning opportunities. In turn this may lead to a more sophisticated and relevant learning contract and substantial, deeper learning.

What Does a Learning Contract Look Like?

Self- and Facilitated Assessment

Begin with helping the student identify what is unique in the setting. Quiz the student about what they are curious about, what puzzles or concerns them in this practice setting. Let them know what type of experiences they can expect and are generally available on a day-to-day basis. If you do not have these already, elicit from the student specified objectives for the placement from the academic curriculum. Ask the student how the self-assessment of their desired learning outcome integrates with the academic curriculum.

Learning Objective

The learning objective clearly states what the learner needs to know, learn or perform. Ensure the learner is realistic and specific about their desired learning within the clinical environment and for themselves.

Action Plan: Learning Strategy

How they will go about learning what it is they need to know or perform?

Evaluation Criteria: Evidence

How will this be revealed to themselves and others? How will the outcome or goal be determined, and by whom? What proof will be offered?

Learning Resources

What resources are required to achieve the objective? Consider such aspects as access to clients or other healthcare professionals, research (evidence-based practice), opportunities to perform particular interventions, methods of recording observations, engagement with information and professional technologies, and access to identified internal or external departments or policies. Guide and support the student through this endeavour.

Target Date for Completion

What timeframe is required to successfully complete the learning objective? Set an explicit time for completion or re-evaluation of the learning to be attained.

Reflections: Evaluation

What personal and professional insights were gained as a result of interacting with the leaning contract? Identify accomplishments. What benefits were gained from completing the learning contract? How will the learner summarise personal insights gleaned from the experience? What challenges did you or the student encounter?

What Now? Setting Future Goals

Having fostered a climate for the learner to achieve their objectives, the teacher may instigate proposals to generate possibilities for creating new learning opportunities. Learners discover, through a process of constructing meaning from learning, their achievements, abilities and areas still requiring improvement for future endeavours.

How will the learner assimilate the new information and intend to use it for future practice? How have they changed? What questions of practice remain unanswered for the learner? What actions need to be taken to extend learning?

Helping the Learner See Meaning: Establishing Learning Goals

Some learners have little insight into their learning needs or may be reluctant to reveal gaps in their knowledge. Others may document little more than the learning objectives already identified in the course or previously achieved. Some global objectives may be attainable in any setting. Objectives need to be specific enough and relevant to the learner, and the current clients and environment need to be meaningful. Your job is to assist the learner to generate new learning from the experience. The next activity considers how you may assist a learner to identify objectives during the time they are with you.

ACTIVITY 4.6

1. Quiz the learner about other knowledge areas they have studied and are studying at present and how they might relate to or inform the proposed learning contract.

2. Inquire about what aspects of the learning environment interest the learner the most. What was it that attracted the learner to the area; the type of clients or the services provided? Use your knowledge of the clinical environment to make suggestions to the learner. Some learners have a lack of knowledge about what the clinical environment has to offer. Offering the learner access to this information may be all it takes to spark their enthusiasm.

3. Anxiety and fear can be a block to learning. Ask the learner if they are apprehensive about any aspect of the forthcoming experience.

4. Ensure the learner knows what is expected of them in the development of the negotiated learning agreement. This might be the learner's first encounter with one.

5. Ask the learner to be specific. Drill into responses to seek further clarification when the objectives are too broad.

6. Help them formulate goals that feature observable behaviour, specific conditions and identified performance, all within an appropriate timeframe.

7. Decide on a starting and end date for the contract.

Learning Contracts

In summary, learning contracts:
- Help learners identify gaps in their knowledge
- Provide an opportunity for the learner to plan their learning and pursue their professional interests

- Alert other staff to the learner's learning requirements
- Act as a communicative link between the learner and clinical teacher
- Engage the learner in meaningful experiences
- Transform learning and the learner.

LEARNING PORTFOLIO DEVELOPMENT

Portfolios are collections of evidence that demonstrate individual learning achievement and document the learning journey (Andre & Heartfield, 2011; Funk, 2007). A portfolio builds a comprehensive picture of the developer's progress and performance in their previous and current experiences. A learning portfolio is intensely personal and takes on the character and idiosyncrasies of its owner. To be effective, portfolios clearly need to be a communicative link with the process and product of the integration of the learner's academic and clinical knowledge (Driessen et al., 2007).

As the teacher, it is not your responsibility to add to the learner's portfolio. Your role is to challenge, question, guide and encourage the learner to discriminate about what to include and how to usefully incorporate evidence to demonstrate their learning and movement towards becoming a competent practitioner. Hrisos, Illing and Burford (2008) indicate that for portfolios to be useful to the learner, support is paramount.

Features of a Portfolio

These days a portfolio can be in the form of a paper-based hard copy, be electronic or a combination. Whatever form it takes, the portfolio remains a personal repository of collected information that can be selectively shared, edited, reflected on and analysed to enhance and demonstrate learning and professional development (Andre & Heartfield, 2011).

Digital and electronic technologies and access to multimedia through Internet hyperlinks has brought the world to the doorstep of clinical practice settings. Today learners, clinicians and teachers are able to access professional and evidence-based practice sites, images, videos, podcasts, online discussions, webinars, blogs and CD-ROMs to inform both practice and learning. The advantage of e-portfolios is that they can be used to record a variety of experiences using text, audio and images, no matter where the clinical experience occurs (Garrett & Jackson, 2006). Familiarity and access to these media require skill and confidence and may challenge both the learner and teacher. It is therefore appropriate to negotiate how the portfolio is developed to demonstrate clearly a degree of confident use and learning potential through an e-portfolio. Whether paper based or electronic, the process and products used to provide evidence of learning in the portfolio are usually structured around four principle categories: artefacts, reproductions, productions and attestations.

Artefacts are materials assembled as part of the learning experience. They are the substance of the way the learner constructs understanding. The type of material students gather may also be an indication of the type of learner they are: visual or auditory, surface or deep, reproductive or transformational. Students may collect information from brochures, practice-area documents developed from within or external to the discipline or from research articles. They may engage with or produce audio or visual recordings, generate questionnaires, conduct research projects, develop client-specific assessments, treatment regimes or educational materials, and engage with an array of electronic resources.

Unlike artefacts, which are learning sources already available to the learner, reproductions portray the personal conceptualisations of the experience of the learner through creative endeavours. Learners may use photography, creative writing—such as poetry, short stories and reflections—and their own artwork such as sketches, diagrams and even cartoons to make explanations and sense of the experience.

Production documents are the essence of the portfolio. Examples of productions may include such items as a learning contract, extracts from journal writings or reflective captions. This sections allows the developer to tell their story of why, how and what worked or went wrong and how they felt about it. In the production category, the learner can display their thoughtful know-how through explanations of the evidence presented. The evidence provides building blocks on which the learner constructs, reflects and reconstructs their knowledge development. Some learners may use concept maps to display how they arrived at particular outcomes. Others can reflectively discern how to use information to inform new situations. Whatever means the learner uses to demonstrate evidence and the process of learning, the production category infuses the portfolio with meaning.

Attestations are evaluative descriptions created by the learner or offered by others that vouch for the authenticity of the specific claims made throughout the portfolio. These can take the form of testimonials, peer reviews, formal assessments and self-appraisals.

Assisting the Learner with a Portfolio Development

The practice setting can generate a diverse range and extraneous amount of 'evidence'. Some learners will gather and hoard an inordinate array of documents and material in an effort to demonstrate their perceived development. There is a danger that the contents of the portfolio can become a cumbersome collection that would be decipherable only to its owner. Conversely, too little information can run the risk of becoming 'sterile', betraying the developer into thinking that they do not require too much evidence to support their learning initiatives. The quality of the portfolio is important because it communicates learning evolution. Too much or little evidence may demonstrate to the teacher the learner's inability to discern relevance and evaluate the worth of material gathered or stored (Andre & Heartfield, 2011).

Managing a Learning Portfolio: What It Could Look Like

Some suggested considerations for creating a learning portfolio are:

1. Determine what form the portfolio will take: paper-based, digital/electronic, online or a multimedia combination.

2. Provide a table of contents or something similar to direct the reader through the portfolio.

3. Ask the learner to provide a statement of purpose for the portfolio: how it relates to their learning contract and the formal objectives of the clinical experience from the academic curriculum.

4. Suggest that the learner write their own statement or philosophy of their discipline, or insert a national or internationally recognised professionally endorsed statement. Propose to the learner that they revisit the statement after the experience to adjust their own statement or acknowledge self-development towards professionally recognised statements.

5. Decide how the portfolio will be reviewed. How will strengths, weaknesses and gaps in evidence be highlighted?

6. Establish what the outcome of the portfolio will be.

7. Determine with the learner strategies to be employed to reflect on and then action learning and professional development as a consequence of the evidence gathered throughout the portfolio.

8. Examples of inclusions may include:
   - Personal philosophical statements
   - Academic placement objectives
   - Learning contract
   - Professional competency statements or standards
   - Clinical assessment forms/tools
   - Client assessments and care management/treatments
   - Case studies
   - Concept maps
   - Journal articles or research reports
   - Websites with explanatory reviews
   - Personal journal or extracts
   - Testimonials
   - Multimedia development and reviews
   - Summary of evidence reports
   - Reflections.

☉ SNAPSHOT

Preparation for learning and teaching experiences is paramount for successful education experiences. This includes developing learning outcomes and lesson plans. Preparation is required for the academic and clinical environments, by both teacher and learner, for integrated experiences. In the clinical environment, boundaries of the experience are negotiated within a welcoming environment and established, open communication.

By creating an environment of support and trust, the teacher is in a unique position to observe the learner's thinking and assist development and progress. Within this atmosphere, the learning experience offers learners the freedom to take safe risks, make choices and provide compelling evidence to generate and demonstrate how they are becoming competent, beginning practitioners.

Preparation for learning acknowledges the importance of the learner who is motivated, self-directed and becoming increasingly self-aware. Strategies identified in this chapter provide the foundation for a mutual undertaking between the learner and teacher in a welcoming environment. The preparative phase, therefore, extends and facilitates the succeeding phases of the learner's experience.

REFERENCES AND FURTHER READING

Anderson, L.W. & Krathwohl, D.R. (Eds). (2001). *A taxonomy for learning, teaching, and assessing: A revision of Bloom's taxonomy of educational objectives.* New York: Longman.

Andre, K. & Heartfield, M. (2011). *Professional portfolios: Evidence of competence for nurses and midwives* (2nd ed.). Sydney: Churchill Livingstone/Elsevier.

Benner, P., Sutphen, M., Leonard, V. & Day, L. (2010). *Educating nurses: A call for radical transformation*. San Francisco: Jossey-Bass.

Billet, S. & Henderson, A. (2011). *Developing learning professionals: Integrating experiences in university and practice settings*. Professional and practice-based learning series. Dordrecht: Springer.

Bloom, B.S. & Krathwohl, D.R. (1956). *Taxonomy of educational objectives: The classification of educational goals, by a committee of college and university examiners*. Handbook I: Cognitive domain. New York: Longmans, Green.

Driessen, E., van Tartwijk J., van der Vleuten, C. & Wass, V. (2007). Portfolios in medical education: Why do they meet with mixed success? A systematic review. *Medical Education*, 41(12): 1224–1233.

Funk, K. (2007). Student experience of learning portfolios in occupational therapy. *Occupational Therapy in Health Care*, 21(1/2): 175–184.

Garrett, B.M. & Jackson, C. (2006). A mobile clinical e-portfolio for nursing and medical students, using wireless personal digital assistants (PDAs). *Nurse Education Today*, 26(8): 647–654.

Hrisos, S., Illing, J.C. & Burford, B. (2008). Portfolio learning for foundation doctors: Early feedback on its use in the clinical workplace. *Medical Education*, 42(2): 214–223.

Janicik, R.W. & Fletcher, K.E. (2003). Teaching at the bedside: A new model. *Medical Teacher*, 25(2): 127–130.

Kennedy-Jones, M. (2005). Contract learning. In M. Rose & D. Best (Eds), *Transforming practice through clinical education, professional supervision and mentoring*. Edinburgh: Elsevier Churchill Livingston.

McAllister, M. (2005). Transformative teaching in nursing education: Preparing for the possible. *Collegian*, 12(1): 13–18.

MacKenzie, L. (2002). Briefing and debriefing of learner fieldwork experiences: Exploring concerns and reflecting on practice. *Australian Occupational Therapy Journal*, 49(2): 82–92.

Papaspyros, S.C., Javangula, K.C., Adluri, R.K. & O'Regan, D.J. (2010). Briefing and debriefing in the cardiac operating room. Analysis of impact on theatre team attitude and patient safety. *Interactive Cardiovascular & Thoracic Surgery*, 10(1): 43–47.

Rose, M. & Best, D. (Eds). (2005). *Transforming practice through clinical education, professional supervision and mentoring*. Edinburgh: Elsevier Churchill Livingstone.

Stockhausen, L. (1994). The clinical learning spiral: A model to develop reflective practitioners. *Nurse Education Today*, 14(3): 363–371.

Stockhausen, L. (1997). The clinical portfolio. *The Australian Electronic Journal of Nursing Education*, 2(2).

Tsang, H.W.H., Paterson, M. & Packer, T. (2002). Self-directed learning in fieldwork education with learning contracts. *British Journal of Therapy and Rehabilitation*, 9(9): 184–189.

CHAPTER 5

Constructing Learning

KEY CONCEPTS

- Large group teaching
- Small group teaching
- Information technologies
- Providing and supporting learning opportunities
- Purposeful observation
- Active demonstration
- Communications

INTRODUCTION

Learners begin to construct their initial knowledge through on-campus learning experiences. Large and small teaching groups are the most common forms of design. Lectures are normally used to convey substantial amounts of information to large groups of learners. In the clinical environment, large and small group teaching may still be used either as part of the clinical experience or for the professional development of employees.

In on-campus experiences, learners commence their rehearsal for professional practice, and the foundation for forthcoming clinical experiences is laid. As learners enter the workplace and participate in the practices of the profession they begin to construct their clinical knowledge. This second phase of constructing learning incorporates the experiences and actual practice that takes place during the practicum.

The construction is located in the learning and the work that is distributed between the learners, the teacher, other members of the discipline and the healthcare team. It is also generally acknowledged that a client's health problem/presentation, diagnosis, interventions, treatments and outcomes provide stimuli for the design and boundaries of clinical educative events. The client's circumstances become the learning situation for learners. Furthermore, engagement in the context and with other health professionals facilitates the development of a professional identity.

This chapter, along with the subsequent chapter, takes into consideration the dimensions of practice as the learner develops procedural knowledge such as: skill acquisition, including cognitive, psychomotor (manual) and attitudes; interpersonal communication development; information usage; and time management. The establishment and maintenance of relationships, especially with the client and staff of the workplace, is also highlighted.

Active participation allows learners to be a part of the actual construction, reinforcement and transformation of professional knowledge. Large and small group teaching differ in their design and the way the teacher and learner interact.

LARGE GROUP TEACHING

For the new teacher, delivering a lecture to groups that can number in the hundreds can be a daunting experience. Likewise, delivering a staff development seminar to groups of peers can also be unsettling for the new teacher. However, considering the way you prepare for teaching encounters will ensure that both the teacher and learners will enjoy the experience. We have already seen in the proceeding chapter that a well-devised lesson plan will assist the process. Here are a few further tips for ensuring the quality of larger-group teaching and improved learning outcomes (Carpenter, 2006):

- Negotiate to sit in on other teachers' classes: you will be surprised at how you can learn to structure different learning events for learners. Other teachers have also developed strategies for engaging learners in novel ways and managing challenging student behaviours or disruptions.
- Use electronic presentation tools such as Powerpoint© sparingly. Identify key concepts or points that you want learners to take away with them from the class. Use learners' ideas and responses and post these on the learning management system. Doing this not only reinforces key concepts but also provides positive reinforcement to the learner.
- Post your presentation notes onto the learning management system prior to the class. This way, learners will not be trying to write continually as they listen.
- Try pod- or vodcasting your session so learners can listen and review the class (anytime, anywhere) (Zanussi et al., 2012; White & Sharma, 2012). This is particularly important for a mature-aged cohort with families or for learners who are employed and find it difficult getting to scheduled classes.

- Variety is the key to fostering motivation, engagement and maintaining interest: develop a 'variety strategy list'. For example:
  - Use short video clips.
  - Pose questions and use hand-held key pad clickers (e.g. Classroom Response Systems) to gauge student responses. The software can instantly tabulate responses, providing feedback to the teacher and learners.
  - Break up the group of learners into smaller groups to engage in investigating or brainstorming a range of ideas regarding a particular topic.
  - Ask another teacher or student to assist you in a role play.
  - Create a range of case-based scenarios that add realism and assist learners to think critically and rehearse clinical reasoning about the topic under discussion.
- Develop a range of strategies to deal with disruptive behaviours. In large classes this might be learners arriving late or continually chatting. Ask the whole group how they would like these behaviours managed.
- Maintain eye contact with learners.
- Redirect learners' questions to other learners. This prompts all learners to engage and avoids relying on the teacher to know everything.
- Conclude the class by providing an overview of the aim of the class and re-visit key concepts and the objectives. Or, have learners reflect and identify their perceived learning outcome from the session. If this class is one in a series of learning events, link it to future sessions. This helps the learner retain important principles and understand how each fits into the bigger picture.
- Take the time to reflect and identify aspects of the class that went well or you will change next time. This should also include reflection on the learning environment and its impact on effective learning outcomes. Evaluate how you will incorporate these reflections into your next class.

- As you become experienced in delivering large group learning events, add to this list. Remember, one day you will be the experienced teacher mentoring the novice.

SMALL GROUP TEACHING

Small group teaching is most often used to complement large group teaching and offers a time for the expansion, exploration, application and reinforcement of concepts and objectives. These groups can be tutorials (face to face or online), laboratory sessions, simulations or clinical placements. For successful small group teaching it is essential to understand group dynamics and the teacher's facilitative role. The role of the teacher is to create an environment that fosters democratic processes to facilitate interaction between learners, for a mutual purpose. There are a number of ways that group processing can be considered by the teacher. One of these is Tuckman's (1965; Tuckman & Jenson, 1977) group formation process.

Originally, Tuckman (1965) nominated that groups work through a four-stage process as they establish themselves and work towards a desired outcome. The stages are: forming, storming, norming and performing. In 1977, this framework (Tuckman & Jensen) was extended to include adjourning. Tuckman believed that, for groups to be successful, they need to work progressively through each of the stages. However, he also indicated that the group may revert to previous stages at periods should the task or individuals in the group require it. Table 5.1 identifies the stages and demonstrates the role the learner and teacher have at each phase.

ACTIVITY 5.1

Investigate Tuckman's stages of group development. Through your reading, discussion with other teachers and your reflections on your engagement with different groups, add to Table 5.1 and record it in your portfolio.

TABLE 5.1 Stages, Roles and Functions: Group Work

Stage	Learner	Facilitator
Forming (orientation)	Enthusiastic and usually has a positive outlook May be anxious about expectations and wonder if they can fulfil their role and get on with the others	Understands that learners tend to need directions to facilitate: • Team-building exercises • Information about the process • Discussion around team roles and responsibilities • Discussion around team norms for working together
Storming (dissatisfaction/ conflict)	Different ideas compete for consideration Members begin to voice their individual differences and concerns in order to feel represented and understood Arguments and subgroups may develop	Accessible, but tends to remain directive in their guidance to facilitate and reinforce group decision making and professional behaviour Reiterates group roles and responsibilities
Norming (resolution/ co-operation)	Differences resolved. Individuals listen to each other, appreciate and support each other, and are prepared to change preconceived views; they feel they are part of a cohesive, effective group Respect, harmony and trust are developing, giving all a sense of self-esteem	Redirects and reminds team of group's ground rules Asks key questions to ensure the group remains on track Ensures all group members are heard

Performing (productivity)	Team members will now feel quite confident, characterised by a state of interdependence and flexibility. Able to work independently. Roles and responsibilities change according to need	Provides praise and reinforcement for achievements
	Group identity, loyalty and morale are all high, and everyone is equally task orientated and people orientated. This high degree of comfort means all of the group's energy can be directed towards the task(s) in hand	
Adjourning (disengaging)	Termination of task behaviours and relationships. Grieving may occur	Provides recognition for participation and achievement

Source: Tuckman & Jensen (1977).

Preparation for Small Group Learning

Before group work commences, ensure learners are aware of the focus of the learning and the educational principles for establishing and using group work. Just as in any other teaching episode, the teacher needs to be prepared. For health professional learners, group work can be discipline-specific or interprofessional. A range of learning resources can initiate, stimulate or structure the aim of the small group work. A few ideas include projects or media to design small group learning events such as: critiquing an article, news report or clinical and evidence-based practice guidelines; examining a particular health policy, book, film, vignette, case study, client or professional scenario;

producing a response to a dilemma; and designing a client-related product (e.g. a device or an education program), a briefing or a reflective debriefing.

Besides understanding the process of group teamwork and structure, the curriculum or purpose for the establishment of the group will determine if the group/s will be self-selecting or designated. Self-selection has both advantages and disadvantages. Often learners will want to work with those whom they know and have an established relationship. Cultural groups also tend to cluster together. However, exposing learners to different types of learners and personalities can assist in the development of teamwork and communicative skills of the whole group.

Establishing Trust

The first step in designing group work is to establish an environment where learners feel safe to express ideas and opinions while protecting their vulnerabilities and maintaining confidentiality.

INSIGHT 5.1

Introductions: Getting to Know One Another

Icebreakers are a non-threatening way for both you and group members to get to know one another. Learners' prior experiences of working in groups will also influence their willingness to engage in group activities. Ask learners about their previous experiences of working in groups: What worked well, and what made it work well? What challenged group work? Was this overcome or left unresolved? What did you learn from this experience?

ACTIVITY 5.2

Investigate a range of icebreakers or group-building exercises you could use. Some group-building activities can also help with developing trust.

Establishing Ground Rules

Following introductions, the teacher can assist learners to develop a team code, group ground rules or guidelines. These serve as a platform for expected group behaviours and processes. Ground rules can be adapted and altered to acknowledge online interactions and be *reviewed several times throughout the projected life of any group* to determine if there is agreement or if a refinement of the principles is required. For example, Schwarz (2002) suggests learners may discuss and decide on:

- What is important and valued by them as a group (e.g. honesty, respecting and valuing one another's ideas and contributions, *only one person speaking at a time, cultural safety and diversity, fair distribution and contribution of tasks,* meeting deadlines, opportunities to discuss, debate and compare understandings with one another [and with the teacher])
- How they will communicate with one another and what communication processes they will use (e.g. Skype, learning management systems [LMS], how often they will meet and record ideas and contributions, how they will manage group emails and documents, and notify in advance of non-attendances)
- How they will deal with such issues as members arriving late to class or meetings, and members not contributing or completing negotiated work on time.

The teacher's role in facilitating small group learning includes:

- *Responsibility*: defining roles, initiating self- and group regulation, respecting diversity
- *Preparation*: prioritising tasks
- *Engagement*: ensuring a democratic group process
- *Focus*: keeping a track of the learners' progress and facilitating time management
- *Productivity/outcomes*: allowing learners to engage in one another's learning and summarise their findings
- *Reflections and actions*: allowing time and ensuring that learners follow up with actions from their engagement with learning from the group activities.

Managing Small Groups

From time to time the teacher will be called upon to help facilitate communication situations that may arise during group work. Some of these are discussed below.

The Talker

'The talker' tries to monopolise the discussion within the group and may also try to dominate the discussion with their point of view (Wheelen, 2013). An approach to this situation is initially to listen, thank them for their ideas, then ask the other group members what they think (ASTD, 2008). You may designate 'the talker' a role as the scribe and have them record the other members' points of view (as their views have already been aired) for summary at the end of the discussion. You may need to stay long enough with the group to ensure 'the talker' does not try to take over the group discussion again. Sitting alongside 'the talker' may also reduce their tendency to dominate the discussion.

The Quiet One

Some group members remain quiet for a number of reasons. 'The quiet one' may be shy, embarrassed to offer their opinion, unprepared for the discussion, or fear ridicule. Using probing questions, invite responses from 'the quiet one'. Give them time to respond, use positive reinforcement and seek further clarifications (ASTD, 2008). As you engage with 'the quiet one', gradually invite others to respond, expanding comments within the group with 'the quiet one'. Once 'the quiet one' gains a little confidence, gradually withdraw and allow the group to ensure all members have a voice.

The Disengaged or the Distractor

Group members can become frustrated when a group member shows disinterest or tries to distract the group from the task at hand. In this situation, call on 'the disengaged or distractor' for specific examples of the topic under discussion (Jaques & Salmon, 2007). Alternatively, pair them with a more positive group member for a brief time to work on a specific aspect of the topic. Have the now 're-engaged and focused one' present their findings to the rest of the group.

The Argumentative One

It is important not to respond to 'the argumentative one' with argument but to acknowledge the person's point of view as valid. Congratulate them and celebrate their point of view and difference, showing the many different ways of perceiving the issue. Invite other group members to identify what 'the argumentative one's' statements add to the discussion and ways to incorporate them into their cognitive or affective schemes. Suggest ways the group can continue productive discussion. You may need to remind the group of their ground rules.

No matter what challenge you or the group are called upon to manage, the most important principle to remember is that all contributions, no matter how good or bad they are, should be valued and used to improve the learning outcomes for all involved.

In review, small group learning:
- Provides a safe haven to explore ideas and skill development
- Helps to consider others' points of view, different ways of looking at concepts and applying theory to various contexts
- Develops self-awareness and appreciation of others' contribution to one's learning
- Provokes inquisitiveness, motivation and engagement
- Allows learners to take responsibility for their own learning
- Develops and changes understanding, attends to feelings, challenges beliefs, values and attitudes
- Extends known to unknown exploration
- Develops ways to work constructively and confidently with others
- Develops oral skills, social interaction and belonging.

Small group teaching may also involve demonstration, simulations, observation or manipulation of professional artefacts of practice. Demonstrations present ways of viewing segments or wholes of practice, whether undertaken by the teacher or the learner. Laboratories and simulations offer a safe environment for a time of rehearsal, discovery, the practising of psychomotor skills, emotional development and preparation for clinical decision making in the workplace.

For the teacher, small group teaching can be compared to conducting an orchestra. As the teacher designs and facilitates learning experiences, they assist the learner to bring pieces of knowledge together, generating cohesion as the learner reformulates their cognitive schemas for knowledge development, preparation and rehearsal for practice.

One-on-One Teaching

One-on-one teaching is the most common form of teaching and learning found in the clinical environment (Gordon, 2003). It is generally thought of in terms of working alongside learners to provide guidance, direction, reinforcement and feedback in context. We have seen throughout this book the many ways that the teacher and the student can engage in clinical educative encounters. The relationship established between the teacher and the learner can be both advantageous and have disadvantages to the learner and the teacher (Fitzgerald, 2011; Grasha, 2002). These are summarised in Table 5.2.

INFORMATION TECHNOLOGIES

Teaching is now well supported with an array of information and communication technologies. Learning management systems (LMS) applications, such as Blackboard© and Moodle©, offer the teacher an assortment of opportunities to 'experiment' with engaging learners. In using online instruction the teacher needs to be mindful of designing learning experiences that assist in addressing the desired

TABLE 5.2 Advantages and Disadvantages of One-on-One Teaching

Advantages	Disadvantages
The Learner	
• Able to identify and have more control over individual learning requirements • Customised individual learning needs can be identified and addressed • Individual attention from the teacher • Feedback is immediate • Fosters progressive achievement and independence • Teacher's expertise can be used as a resource	• May feel overwhelmed and anxious as practices are more intensely scrutinised • Teacher can take over • Too much teacher support can foster learned helplessness • Can try to live up to the teacher's unrealistic expectations • Teacher can become overly directive, explaining too much
The Teacher	
• Better understanding of the learner's individual needs • Teaching can be tailored to meet the learner's requirements • A variety of teaching methods can be used such as role modelling, observations and demonstrations • Initial assessment and ongoing evaluation • Observation of all learning domains is possible • Helps learners explore options in practice as they arise • Can explain thought processes as situations unfold	• Individual learning differences not taken into account • Can 'clone' learners in the teacher's own image • Can misjudge learner's abilities and readiness to undertake more autonomous roles and tasks • Can be time consuming • Unsure and unprepared learners can be dependent upon the teacher, or monopolise their time at the expense of other learners or clients

learning outcomes. Learners' different learning styles can also be accommodated by designing a variety of activities.

With the range of interactive tools now available, teaching can take on new dimensions. Learning management systems facilitate the posting of course outlines, lecture notes, assessment tasks and notices to learners on electronic bulletin boards. Online interactive activities can also be incorporated such as pod- or vodcasts, short visual clips, pre- and post-test material; and chat rooms, blogs or online discussion groups can be used to pose or answer student questions. Learners are able to discuss clinical and academic scenarios, reflect on their experiences and interact with or without the lecturer (Tan, Ladyshewsky & Gardner, 2010).

Electronic and mobile learning are proving to be useful 'anytime, anywhere' rapid-access tools for learning and assessment. Taylor et al. (2010) indicate that mobile learning improves teacher and peer interactions and real-time access to information, feedback and contextualised reflection. Learners and teachers have rapid access to a range of useful web resources to inform queries in practice and to assist ongoing learning (Jeffrey & Bourgeois, 2011). Furthermore, interactive tools have the interesting outcome of helping learners at a distance achieve a sense of belonging and connection to fellow learners.

The teacher is also able to note the number and quality of the interactions and provide assistance as required. The use of technology for clinical assignments can also assist learners to become more discriminating in the use of evidence and how technology can support learning and appropriate client outcomes. However, it should be remembered that learners are not just learning through technology. Teachers are assisting learners to know how to use and manipulate knowledge, how to use information and communication technology; they are showing them how this can benefit their future practice as a health professional.

In the Clinical Environment

The clinical experience is viewed from a perspective of 'complete-ness' (of beginning, middle and end). Observation of the learner during this phase is crucial because reflections, between the observer and the observed, can heighten the experience and reveal different perspectives of the same experience. Demonstrations by the teacher or practice partner, with accompanying commentary, further assist learners to understand how knowledge and skills are integrated to construct the work of the discipline and aid learner's dexterity, acqui-sition, retention and competence.

From time to time such factors as directing, communicating, enhancing clinical reasoning, the client, other professionals and the context will influence this phase of learner development.

PROVIDING AND SUPPORTING LEARNING OPPORTUNITIES

Teachers in practice contexts are alert to learning opportunities that are planned as well as often unplanned as client presentations and clinical events unfold in practice. To assist learners to partici-pate and construct their beginning practice, the learning supports that teachers use are purposeful observation, active demonstration, sharing information, making suggestions and fostering self-reliance. As the teacher demonstrates competence, they combine learning opportunities with the duality of caring and managing clients, a relationship that exposes sophisticated teaching strategies.

Teachers in practice display or role model in action, to reinforce that more than technical competence is required to provide competent care and client management. The routine procedures required in everyday work induct learners into the ways of coming to know and understand their professional roles and identity, the client and their management, so they are not just tasks.

Teachers do this by using verbal and non-verbal forms of communication. These communications carry the language, science, art and culture of the health discipline. Observational, linguistic and demonstrative exchanges provide information but, more importantly, they transfer the cultural and experiential knowledge necessary for induction into the culture of practice. The exposition and practice within a given context are concomitant.

INSIGHT 5.2

All health professionals conduct themselves using an ethical framework for professional practice. Whether observations or demonstrations are used, ethical behaviour is essential. Permission needs to be sought from all involved. Judgements need to be suspended, and privacy and confidentiality assured. Sensitivity and respect for the client, their culture and professional boundaries are also required.

ACTIVITY 5.3

Consider and make a list of each of the ethical behaviours used during observations or demonstrations. Use this information to provide a step in planning every supportive learning opportunity. This is also a useful exercise to consider for interprofessional observations and demonstrations. Talk with other health professionals (from your discipline and others) and discuss what they find challenging or stressful while being observed by others or demonstrating. Collaboratively, identify ways to promote personal and professional safety and break down professional barriers.

PURPOSEFUL OBSERVATIONS

Health professionals are skilled observers and there is much to be observed in the clinical environment. For the learner, understanding what, who, how and why experienced practitioners notice, through observation within their practice, can be a daunting and complex activity. Therefore, the purpose of observations in clinical practice environments is crucial. It is looking with purpose. The ability to view clinical events analytically and critically is acquired through the recognition, interpretation and encoding of everyday events and interactions. It develops an understanding of the variety of perspectives in most situations.

Observation becomes a time for the learner to use different lenses. The learner watches and notices both familiar and unfamiliar segments or the whole overall environment: professional skills, behaviours, client reactions and situations. Observations also assist the learner to develop an ability to be discerning about what they see.

The focus of the observation will vary depending on the situation and who is involved. Defining the scope of the observation will assist the learner to take notice of the smaller segments (focus points) encompassing a complete episode. These observations can be structured or unstructured. Structured observations provide a framework for the learner. Unstructured observations may be used to develop a wide-view panorama of an activity or event. Encourage learners to consider the broader context in which they are observing, not only the aspects related to the specific client and their care. No matter how the observations are determined, the desired outcome is the same: to gain insights and promote meaning making and relevance (see Table 5.3).

TABLE 5.3 Benefits of Purposeful Observations in the Clinical Setting

- Allow recognition, interpretation, analysis and evaluation of events
- Aid development of understanding
- Allow identification of familiar and unfamiliar aspects
- Assist development of discerning abilities
- Facilitate focus
- Allow for gaining insight
- Promote making meaning and relevance

Observation Schedule: Understanding Roles

Negotiating with the learner what is to be observed and how observations will be carried out will ensure that the focus and parameters are defined. The observations should be relevant to the learning requirements identified by the learner, defined by the curriculum and available within the clinical setting.

Defining each other's role, that of learner and teacher, for forthcoming observations, ensures that each participant is aware of the other's involvement. Clarification of observer roles can lessen misinterpretation. This can deflect anxiety and ensure the safety of the learner and client. It can ease tension and heighten awareness.

The teacher can offer to be a benevolent presence, directly observe the learner with or without verbal or intervention cues, or indirectly make observations from a distance. Likewise, the learner can be a participant in the observation, be observed, be a spectator with or without discussion, or engage in covert surveillance. There is a fine balance for the clinical teacher and the learner between hovering and intrusion and unobtrusive, sensitive involvement (Keating, Dalton & Davidson, 2009).

ACTIVITY 5.4

1. With your discipline colleagues, prepare an observation schedule based on your role. What aspects of your role would you consider essential for the learner entering your work environment to notice?

2. Develop an observational schedule of a key skill crucial to your work environment. Consider what you would include and why.

3. In tandem with a learner, develop an observational schedule of a practice area the learner identified in their learning contract. This activity is an excellent time to negotiate the specific aspects to be observed and clarify the expectations of each other. The observational schedule is also an ideal tool to assist with assessment, reflection and feedback.

Making Observations

Observations of other learners or health professionals in the clinical setting allow learners to view how perspectives on a similar event can vary. The perceptions and recall of how others react and respond to specific situations help the learner to make comparisons and consider variations to practice. Images of practice facilitate the learner's acceptance or rejections of aspects of the activity being viewed. Observations are also powerful tools for the learner to affirm their construction of professional identity, ethical and cultural practices. Such considerations provide key prompts for reflective exercises and collegial dialogue. Observations of professional roles, responsibilities and functions within multidisciplinary healthcare environments can also extend the learner's perceptual view.

In the various clinical environments that learners enter, the observations they make and are involved with include:

- Learners observing the teacher: for revealing momentary reactions and responses
- Teachers observing learners: this is for improving learning and assessment
- Learners observing the client
- Clients observing learners
- Learners observing one another; peer observations
- Learners observing other members of their discipline in different roles
- Learners observing other health professionals
- Learners observing their surrounding environment (local and global, geographical, social, political and economic).

These variations are discussed below.

Learners Observing the Teacher

Learners often indicate that, prior to being observed themselves, they wish to observe the teacher or practice partner in a similar situation. This assists the learner to see how a experienced practitioner deals with not just the segment under observation but how this is incorporated into the overall professional context and/or management of the client. As the teacher is observed in practice, they make momentary reactions and responses that may extenuate from the unpredictable nature of their practice. As the learner makes these observations, they see how the rehearsal of the practice can be enacted and may also unconsciously absorb how the experienced practitioner deals with not just everyday events but models expert practices (Stockhausen, 2006).

Teachers Observing Learners

Teachers spend extended and significant amounts of time observing learners carrying out a diverse range of professional activities. Observation of learners can be used as both a teaching strategy or to assess the learner. In supporting learning through observations, teachers and practice partners provide information and suggestions on practical matters so that learners can refine their beginning practices.

A characteristic that often occurs when teachers observe learners (and demonstrate) is that of 'talk through' (Stockhausen, 2000). Talk through can be defined as the verbal cues and directions made by the teacher as a learner performs a particular activity. Talk through is usually supported by locatives (here, there), demonstratives (this, that) and such verbs as put, tilt or look. If these utterances were separated from the context in which they occurred, they would be ambiguous. However, as part of the observation, the talk through takes on contextual significance for the learner. These verbal cues introduce learners to nuances and variations on ways of practice (Stockhausen, 2000). However, caution is also required to ensure the teacher does not continually direct the learner on what to do and how. It is vital that the learner has time to think and make decisions for themselves (Facione, 2005).

Positive encouragement usually accompanies talk through and it reinforces the learner's attempts. In offering information and constructive support, the teacher motivates the learner to strive for success. Furthermore, praise should be appropriate and varied to ensure sincerity and genuine regard.

Next time you directly observe a learner, think about the verbal cues you use to direct their attention to specific details about the activity. Think about how these cues can be expanded upon to add contextual information and further explanation.

Observing the learner for assessment purposes is discussed in more detail in Chapter 7.

Learners Observing Clients

Observation of the client is fundamental to data collection and the interpretive skills used by all health professionals. Through observation health professionals notice and interpret a complex array of non-verbal communication. These non-verbal observations can be compared with or validated against other objective client data. The client observations can be specific or detailed. Collectively these observations can create an in-depth collage of the client.

The types of direct non-verbal observations health professionals make of clients include:

- Facial expressions or grimaces
- Eye contact
- Responses to investigations, pain or treatments
- Posture and gait
- Physical attributes and characteristics
- Gestures
- Interaction with the environment.

There are multiple observations of the client that a learner could make in the clinical or social environment. Some health professionals have the opportunity to view practice and client interactions through observational rooms. Other health professionals may have access to various methods to observe interactions, such as video conferencing.

Clients Observing Learners

Clients are in a prime position to observe learners either as participants in experiences or as detached observers (Stockhausen, 2009). Seeking feedback from clients can be a useful tool for the teacher. Often a client can make different, but very valuable, observations of the learner from those of the teacher. In seeking client interpretations of their observations, the teacher is advised also to pursue other objective data to support the client's views. Responses to treatments and other client variables may distort a client's perceptions. The section on demonstrations in this chapter further highlights ways in which clients participate in learning experiences.

Learners Observing One Another: Peer Observations

Many health professionals use peer observation and learning to support learner activities in practice settings (Rose & Best, 2005). If peer observations are to be used as a teaching and learning strategy, the teacher should gain consent from the learners and determine the overall purpose of the peer observation.

As learners observe one another or work together, they engage in a supportive and encouraging collaboration (Secomb, 2008). The use of peers as role models has been argued as powerful for learners (Nestel & Kidd, 2005). A sense of security of not being alone in unfamiliar activities often prevails. Learners have comprehensive knowledge of their formal curricula, professional ideals, or what has been taught and is expected to be known. This can provide learners with a common point to observe, critique, interpret, reflect on and improve one another's practices. Indeed, as early as 1964, Piaget (in DeLisi & Golbeck, 1999) postulated that co-operative learning and peer tutoring can initiate thought processes. The process of formulating thoughts in order to express them to others can facilitate metacognitive development and be shared between learners.

Having learners identify what they know and what gaps in knowledge or cues they learned from one another can provide a stimulus for learning self-regulation and a trigger for small group work and debriefing sessions. As the teacher interacts with the peers they can provide feedback and offer to extend the ideas expressed, thus reinforcing peer-generated thought processes and knowledge.

The teacher also needs to be mindful of different developmental levels of learners within the same group. The more advanced peer may be able to assist the less able learner but become frustrated and disengage if this is abused. However, the less able learner may feel anxious about being observed or questioned about their practices. An experienced learner entering a new specialty field of practice may also experience anxiety but be expected to be competent.

Teachers can promote peer learning as a supportive interaction that assists with building professional identity, performance review confidence and team approaches to care and client management. All health professionals need to work together. Having learners observe both members of their own discipline (community of practitioners) and other healthcare professionals highlights the necessity for interprofessional communication to ensure appropriate client outcomes. Through these observations, learners take note of how professionals interact, respect one another, model appropriate behaviours, and collaborate and consult. Interactions between other health professionals and the teacher can also demonstrate collaborative problem solving and intervention. Consultation and collaboration with others and one another also extends personal and professional courtesy and knowledge to provide quality care. Confidential professional conversations with other health professionals can take place formally or casually.

Learners Observing Other Members of Their Discipline

Learners not only spend time observing the teacher or practice partner but they also observe other members within the community of practice. There are any number of observations that the learner can make within their own discipline. The way in which professionals communicate traverses all health disciplines.

Not everyone works in the same way and learners can observe how different practitioners apply and adapt theoretical constructions of the profession to individual client and contextual situations. These types of observations provoke inquisitiveness and, with multiple observations, learners begin to develop a deeper understanding of how members of a profession enact, reproduce and co-produce their culture of practice.

Furthermore, within each health discipline, professional roles have expanded and specialties developed. Observing these professional specialists also assists the learner to view how these roles contribute to the client's care and management.

Learners Observing Other Health Professionals

As learners observe other healthcare professionals they develop an appreciation of other healthcare discipline roles and responsibilities. Furthermore, Zarezadeh, Pearson & Dickinson (2009, p. 5) believe that interprofessional learning creates 'a more positive approach to others, trust among professions, mutual respect and understanding, opening lines of communications, creating opportunities to learn from and about others'. Learners also observe and become privy to how other healthcare professionals contribute to the client's care management (Booth et al., 2001). Learners gain insights into interdisciplinary co-operation. The learner begins to 'see' comparisons in professional clinical reasoning and co-construction of knowledge (Zarezadeh, Pearson & Dickinson, 2009). This is often seen at client case conferences or 'rounds'.

ACTIVITY 5.5

After seeking permission, have a learner sit in on a client case conference and ask them to observe and listen to how each health professional contributes. Focus the observation on one or two aspects. Some examples may include communication styles, the client information presented, how decisions are made and by whom, and how outcomes were reached.

Learners Observing Their Environment

We often take for granted the location of where we work (Green et al., 2008). The way practitioners work in specific environments is highlighted by their ability to adapt to local conditions. This is particularly shown in the way practices are adjusted in metropolitan, urban, rural or remote locations, hospitals, clinics, community organisations or the client's home. While geographical location will influence the way we practice, other contextual factors may equally affect the way we learn and work.

The client, learner and teacher cannot be separated from their environment. Each participant brings to each encounter their own particular life circumstances that influence their healthcare. To actually 'see' this may be difficult. Discovering how our own and the client's social, political and economic background, age, gender, ethnicity and culture can impact on the way healthcare is accessed and delivered, can alert health professionals to examine the judgements made about clients and to question equity and social justice issues related to healthcare (Benner et al., 2010).

Learners are also encouraged to observe the way health professionals work within sustainability practices through their access and use of equipment and resources.

INSIGHT 5.4

Within different practice settings the learner can use visual accounts of practice and active discourse to:

- Direct attention to salient features under observation
- Make descriptions of practice, interactions and settings
- Visualise; form images of practice
- Make comparisons
- Focus attention
- Ease fears

- Form opinions

- Judge progress.

ACTIVE DEMONSTRATION

Demonstrations extend observational teaching methods. They provide a three-dimensional and multisensory example of professional practice. Demonstrations can illustrate how to perform a procedure or skill, use and manipulate equipment, respond to situations and how to display appropriate interactions with clients and others. Most demonstrations have three components to them: a demonstration by a person experienced in the procedure, followed by a return demonstration by the learner where the teacher supervises, with the final phase seeing the learner confident to undertake the procedure independently.

There is inconsistency in the literature about when explanations should be made during demonstrations (Rose & Best, 2005). Suggestions are that the demonstration should be performed without explanation in the first instance, with increasing dialogue by either the teacher or learner as the procedure is performed again.

Repeating part of or the whole procedure aids retention. This works well in the simulated learning environment or for the manipulation of technical equipment, but when the client or others are involved, the demonstration can become 'sterile' and lack spontaneity, surprise and inquisitiveness. The client may also feel that their presence is of little consequence.

Contextualising the demonstration is important, for what works in one situation may not always be possible in another. While certain aspects of professional skills have similarities, the learner needs to be alerted to the principles governing the client's specific condition, management and environment, and be able to adapt to different situations, at different times and to client idiosyncrasies.

Getting Started: Guiding Principles

Before you demonstrate a professional activity to the learner:
- Seek permission from the client
- Establish the relevance and purpose
- Negotiate the distributed involvement
- Prepare all involved
- Ensure all equipment and resources are functional and available
- Ensure you have time
- Prior to its commencement, briefly explain the activity to the learner
- Ensure the learner has a clear view
- Know what you are doing!
- Make connections between theoretical and client presentation
- Prepare to reflect upon the activity and provide feedback.

Demonstrations can be performed with or without the client, depending on the situation and what is being demonstrated. There is a range of active demonstrations modelled by various contributors within the clinical learning environment. This section presents three. The first is conducted by the teacher, the second is carried out by the learner, and the third is facilitated by clients.

Teacher Demonstrations

A demonstration by the teacher provides the learner with an action-orientated display of how a procedure or interaction appears in practice. Demonstrations of this nature allow learners to observe the teacher undertaking activities of practice. Many learners have had an opportunity to practise a professional activity only in the controlled university environment or laboratory prior to entering a practice setting. Before a learner proceeds to tackle a newly acquired skill, they often ask to observe the teacher or practice partner first. This gives the learners a panorama of the activity within a broader context.

As the teacher performs the activity, it gives learners an opportunity to observe and question variations in actions and client responses. Interestingly, although demonstrations of a technical skill may be requested by the learner or suggested by the teacher or practice partner, the actual demonstration often goes well beyond the bounds of just the technical aspects of a skill. Stalmeijer et al.'s (2009) study found that medical students appreciated clinicians who explained why and how they performed procedures in certain ways. The client and the situation also add to variations and conditions under which a technical skill can be demonstrated. Thus teaching and learning occur in the moments they are being demonstrated. Table 5.4 summarises the benefits of active teacher demonstration.

Demonstrations by Learners

It is unfair to expect the learner's first attempts to be perfect. They require time to practise and adjust to situations and clients. The teacher also needs to make judgements about the learner's state of readiness, their grasp of underpinning theory and ability to undertake the task. These judgements are crucial to ensuring the learner receives an appropriate level of challenge and support. Client safety is paramount as learners demonstrate tasks.

Beginning learners have a tendency to focus on one segment of an activity at a time. In the complex clinical environment the learner may not be able to grasp whole situations. This suggests that, until mastery of the smaller unit and confidence undertaking the activity is achieved, the learner may not be able to move onto or grasp whole situations. It may also be difficult for the learner to be aware of the client's responses. The teacher needs to be mindful of all aspects of

---

TABLE 5.4 Benefits of Active Demonstration

- Illustrates how to perform a skill, manipulate equipment, respond to a certain situation
- Role models appropriate interactions
- Allows repetition to aid retention
- Allows for the identification of principles governing practice
- Enables procedures to be broken down into smaller components

skill acquisition and ensure that the learner is alerted to the overall event and not just the technical components.

ACTIVITY 5.6

Investigate and determine the appropriate steps required for an active demonstration. This process can be used to develop a checklist for any specific skill considered necessary to expose competent practice in the clinical setting.

Develop a checklist of an interdisciplinary procedural skill. Hand washing is a good example because all health professionals are required to perform it! There are likely to be several published criteria or checklists from various health disciplines. All will be based on the governing principles of infection prevention and management. Consult at least three; make comparisons and develop your own checklist for your specific clinical area.

Client Involvement in Learning

Clients are usually willing to participate in the learner's skill development to assist them in gaining experience and moving towards becoming qualified (Wykurz & Kelly, 2002). Clients also find satisfaction in helping learners and are a source of information, encouragement and feedback for the learner (Stockhausen, 2009). In their model for effective, ethical bedside teaching, Janicik and Fletcher (2003) argue for seeking permission from the client well prior to the encounter, empowering them to have control of the experience. This also facilitates establishing the role that the client will play. Sayed-Hassan et al. (2012) also remind clinical teachers and learners to ensure respect and dignity of clients in any educational encounters.

As participants in the learner's experience, clients believe that learners can gain firsthand knowledge of the client's experience from their perspective (Lathlean et al., 2006). This stance is expounded by Spencer et al. (2000, p. 853), as they believe clients 'see themselves as experts in their own condition (both in terms of telling and showing), as exemplars of the condition (intuitively, perhaps, recognizing the importance of "illness scripts"), and as having a hand in the development of professional skills and attitudes'. Furthermore, Bleakly & Bligh (2008) consider that, through dialogue, the client co-produces knowledge with medical students, assisting the student to understand more fully their role and the client's health experience.

Clients involved in teaching and learning are willing demonstrators of how they have adapted to aspects of their condition and manipulate their self-care and management. Others are willing to assist in curriculum development, ensuring the health consumer's voice is incorporated (McAllister, 2005).

Including Clients in Teaching Interactions

Incorporate the following suggestions in client–learner interactions:

- Collaborate with clients to produce learning materials that provide accounts of their health experience.
- Have clients demonstrate, to the learner, how they perform certain tasks familiar to them. An example may be a person with diabetes who administers their own insulin. Clients can explicate the emotional or subjective dimensions of their health experience, assisting the learner to understand different perspectives of health events.
- Detailed interviews with clients can delve into socio-cultural aspects of their health experiences that can then be used as triggers for more rigorous investigation.
- Some clients are willing to tell their unscripted or scripted health experience story. The teacher can assist the client to present (teach) their story to individuals or groups of learners and help the client prepare for questions the learners may ask.
- Sessions or interviews with clients can be recorded for future screening.

- Ask the client how they perceived the learner interacted with them. Did the student ask questions that provoked ideas or responses not previously considered by the client?
- Did the learner seek information from the client on how they manage their condition or situation?
- Was the learner able to incorporate the client's ideas to manage their care?
- Did the client consider the learner was able to understand their condition or empathise with their situation?
- Ask the client if or how the learner was able to offer constructive ideas to facilitate self-management.
- Ask the client what observations they made of the learner.
- Ask the client what they learnt from their encounter with the learner.

INSIGHT 5.5

As clients interact with the learner they become accidental teachers and often broker educative experiences. They become the originator and the mediator through which teaching and learning moments occur between themselves, the learner and clinical teacher (Stockhausen, 2009).

ACTIVITY 5.7

Identify how you ethically and actively involve the client in the learning experience.

Investigate how you can involve the client more constructively in active observations, interactions or demonstrations to help teach the learner.

Consider how you can use this information to empower clients to support the learner's knowledge development.

Through authentic encounters with clients, learners 'connect' with the client in a sensitive way. Learners gain knowledge of how to respond, interpret and collect signals from the client. As they do this, the student gathers a range of cues to offer information, not only during the initial encounter, but as exemplars for future practice.

Supporting Learning through Communication

Health professionals use a complex array of verbal and non-verbal communication during their practice. Each chapter throughout this book is interspersed with multiple ways that professionals, including learners, communicate with one another. Through verbal communication we not only talk about the client, their condition, presentations, interventions and management but the language of the profession is spoken within and also passed onto the next generation of professionals.

INSIGHT 5.6

To the neophyte or new employee entering the clinical environment, professional acronyms and jargon used can be alienating. The language we use can be alienating, or be used as a learning episode. Think about the professional language you use in your everyday encounters with members of your profession. Imagine you are a learner observing and listening to these professional exchanges. What would be your reaction?

How do you ensure that 'profession speak' does not become a barrier to learning for the newcomer in the community of practitioners?

How do you invite and aid the learner to include them in professional exchanges?

Documentation

All health professionals use various forms of documentation to communicate and record a range of investigations that inform assessment and identity problems, diagnosis, interventions, treatments, progress and responses. The different forms of documentation, and the way they can be incorporated to support learners' learning, can be powerful tools for the teacher. Documentation can be paper-based or electronic.

The use of technology, particularly mobile technologies such as personal digital assistants (PDAs), desktop computers and integrated management systems, can support clinical decision making and client data organisation. According to Farrell (2009) and other researchers (Staudinger, Höß & Ostermann, 2009), technology as a new communication medium supports learning in clinical environments by providing valuable access to point-of-contact information in real time. Computerised technologies can record a variety of information on the client for the learner and for the evaluative monitoring of the learner by the teacher.

New computerised technologies provide a comprehensive repository for client clinical data. Learners have the potential to access and retrieve computerised client records. Information for learning purposes can include client histories, medical images (x-rays, scans), diagnostics (pathology results, reports) and surveillance images. Learners are also able to access expert resources and information, including evidence-based practice databases. Pre-loaded learning and assessment materials can also assist the learner to traverse academic knowledge and clinical and client presentations (Kho et al., 2006). Monitoring for quality assessment, risk management and health and disease statistics provides useful information for the more advanced learner.

INSIGHT 5.7

There is a vast amount of information available to learners. With the range of documented resources and computerised technologies used in the workplace, the learner can be overwhelmed with what to access and how to use it. The teacher can assist the learner to become discerning with what information to use for knowledge development and making clinical decisions.

ACTIVITY 5.8

Identify what computerised technologies are used in your clinical setting.

How do you integrate documentation and computerised technologies into the learning experience of the learner?

What type of information do you or the learner access to assist learning?

How do learners engage with the technologies available to them to support their learning?

How do they use this information to add to their repertoire to assist their clinical decision making?

How do you gauge the success by which the documentation is used to support the student's learning?

Use the answers to the above questions to design a clinical scenario that will assist the learner with integrating client information and the computerised technologies used to assist their clinical decision making.

📷 SNAPSHOT

As learners engage in the practice disciplines of specific clinical environments, they begin to piece together how to participate in and construct their discipline knowledge and identity. The principal learning and teaching strategies used to facilitate and support this transition are purposeful observations and active demonstrations. The fostering of learning episodes hinges on interpersonal and communicative endeavours and exchanges.

In the subsequent chapter, learning supports are extended. The teacher and more-experienced practitioner draw upon discipline knowledge, expertise and experience to assist the learner to build upon their involvement in the discipline and to reconstruct their beginning knowledge or extended understandings of their profession.

REFERENCES

American Society for Training & Development (ASTD) (Eds). (2008). *10 steps to successful facilitation*. Alexandria, VA: American Society for Training & Development. Available via www.astd.org.

Azer, S. (2005). Challenges facing PBL tutors: 12 tips for successful group facilitation. *Medical Teacher*, 27(8): 676–681.

Benner, P., Stuphen, M., Leonard, V. & Day, L. (2010). *Educating nurses: A call for radical transformation*. San Francisco: Jossey-Bass.

Bleakly, A. & Bligh, J. (2008). Students learning from patients: Let's get real in medical education. *Advances in Health Sciences Education*, 13(1): 89–107.

Booth, J., Davidson, I., Winstanley, J. & Waters, K. (2001). Observing washing and dressing of stroke patients: Nursing intervention compared with occupational therapists. What is the difference? *Journal of Advanced Nursing*, 33(1): 98–105.

Carpenter, J.M. (2006). Effective teaching methods for large classes. *Journal of Family & Consumer Sciences Education*, 24(2): 13–23.

DeLisi, R. & Golbeck, S. (1999). Implications of Piagetian theory for peer learning. In A. O'Donnell & A. King (Eds), *Cognitive perspectives on peer learning* (pp. 3–37). Mahwah, NJ: Lawrence Erlbaum Associates.

Facione, P. (2005). Critical thinking: What it is and why it counts. Keynote address presented at the 2nd Ministry of Health International Nursing Conference and 10th Joint Singapore–Malaysian Nursing Conference, Singapore.

Farrell, M.J. (2009). Use of handheld computers in nursing education. In B. Staudinger, V. Höß & H. Ostermann (Eds), *Nursing and clinical informatics: Socio-technical approaches* (pp. 239–252). Hershy, PA: IGI Global (online). Doi: 10.4018/978-1-60566-234-3.

Fitzgerald, K. (2011). Instructional methods and settings. In S. Bastable, P. Gramet, S. Jacobs & D. Sopczyk (Eds), *Health professional educator: Principles of teaching and learning*. Sudbury, MA: James and Bartlett Learning.

Fujishin, R. (2007). *Creating effective groups: The art of small group communication* (2nd ed.). Lanham, MD: Rowman & Littlefield.

Gordon, J. (2003). ABC of learning and teaching in medicine: One to one teaching and feedback. *British Medical Journal* (clinical research ed.), 326(7388): 543–535.

Grasha, A. (2002). The dynamics of one-on-one teaching. *College Teaching*, 50(4): 139–146.

Green, R., Gregory, R. & Mason, R. (2009). Preparing social work practice in diverse contexts: Introducing an integrated model for class discussion. *Social Work Education: International Journal*, 28(4): 413–422.

Henry, P. (2006). Making groups work in the classroom. *Nurse Educator*, 31(1): 26–30.

Janicik, R. & Fletcher, K. (2003). Teaching at the bedside: A new model. *Medical Teacher*, 25(2): 127–130.

Jaques, D. (2003). ABC of learning and teaching in medicine: Teaching small groups. *British Medical Journal*, 326(7387): 492–494.

Jaques, D. & Salmon, G. (2007). *Learning in groups: A handbook for face-to-face and online environments*. London: Routledge.

Jeffrey, K. & Bourgeois, S. (2011). The effect of personal digital assistants in supporting the development of clinical reasoning in undergraduate nursing students: A systematic review. *Joanna Briggs Institute Library of Systematic Reviews*, 9(2): 38–68.

Kenny, R., Park, C., Van Neste-Kenny, J., Burton, P. & Meiers, J. (2009). Using mobile learning to enhance the quality of nursing practice education. In M. Ally (Ed.), *Mobile Learning Transforming the Delivery of Education and Training*. Athabasca University, Edmonton, Canada: AU Press.

Keating, J., Dalton, M. & Davidson, M. (2009). Assessment in clinical education. In C. Delaney & E. Molloy (Eds), *Clinical education: Evidence, practice and understanding* (pp. 147–172). Sydney: Elsevier.

Kho, A., Henderson, L.E., Dressler, D.D. & Kripalani, S. (2006). Use of handheld computers in medical education. *Journal of General Internal Medicine*, 21(5): 531–537.

Lathlean, J., Burgess, A., Coldham, T., Gibson, C., Herbert, L., Levett-Jones, T., Simons, L. & Tee, S. (2006). Experiences of service users and care participation in healthcare education. *Nurse Education in Practice*, 6(6): 424–429.

McAllister, M. (2005). Transformative teaching in nursing education: Leading by example. *Collegian*, 12(2): 11–16.

McKimm, J. (2009). Small group teaching. *British Journal of Hospital Medicine*, 70(11): 654–657.

Nestel, D. & Kidd, J. (2005). Peer assisted learning in patient centred interviewing: The impact on student tutors. *Medical Teacher*, 27(5): 439–444.

Rose, M. & Best, D. (Eds). (2005). *Transforming practice through clinical education, professional supervision and mentoring*. Edinburgh: Elsevier Churchill Livingston.

Sayed-Hassan, R., Bashour, H. & Koudsi, A. (2012). Patient attitudes towards medical learners at Damascus University teaching hospitals. *BMC Medical Education*, 12: 13.

Schiola, S. (2011). *Making group work easy: The art of successful facilitation*. Portland, OR: Rowman & Littlefield Education.

Schwarz, R. (2002). *The skilled facilitator: A comprehensive resource for consultants, facilitators, managers, trainers and coaches* (2nd ed.). San Francisco: Jossey-Bass.

Schwarz, R., Davidson, A., Carlson, P. & McKinney, S. (2005). *The skilled facilitator fieldbook: Tips, tools, and tested methods for consultants, facilitators, managers, trainers, and coaches*. San Francisco: Jossey-Bass.

Secomb, J. (2008). A systematic review of peer teaching and learning in clinical education. *Journal of Clinical Nursing*, 17(6): 703–716.

Spencer, J., Blackmore, D., Heard, S., McCorie, P., McHaffie, D., Scherpbier, A., Tarum, S., Singh, K. & Southgate, L. (2000). Patient-orientated learning: A review of the role of the patient in the education of medical students. *Medical Education*, 34(10): 851–857.

Stacy, R. & Spencer, J. (1999). Patients as teachers: A qualitative study of patients' views on their role in a community based undergraduate project. *Medical Education*, 33(9): 688–694.

Stalmeijer, R., Dolmans, D., Wolfhagen, I. & Scherpbier, A. (2009). Cognitive apprenticeship in clinical practice: Can it stimulate learning in the opinion of students? *Advances in Health Sciences Education*, 14(4): 535–546.

Staudinger, B., Höß, V. & Ostermann, H. (2009). *Nursing and clinical informatics: socio-technical approaches*. Hershy, PA: IGI Global (online). Doi: 10.4018/978-1-60566-234-3.

Stockhausen, L. (2000). The teaching and learning of nursing: Perspectives of registered nurses and students. PhD thesis, University of Queensland.

Stockhausen, L. (2006). Métier artistry: Revealing reflection in action in everyday practice. *Nurse Education Today*, 26(1): 54–62.

Stockhausen, L. (2009). The patient as experience broker in clinical learning: Nurse education in practice. *Nurse Education Today*, 9(3): 184–189.

Suikkala, A. & Leino-Kilpi, H. (2005). Nursing student–patient relationship: Experiences of students and patients. *Nurse Education Today*, 25(5): 344–354.

Tan, S., Ladyshewsky, R. & Gardner, P. (2010). Using blogging to promote clinical reasoning and metacognition in undergraduate physiotherapy fieldwork programs. *Australasian Journal of Educational Technology*, 26(3): 355–368.

Taylor, J.D., Dearnley, C., Laxton, J., Coates, C., Treasure-Jones, T., Campbell, R. & Hall, I. (2010). Developing a mobile learning solution for health and social care practice. *Distance Education*, 31(2): 175–192.

Tuckman, B. (1965). Developmental sequence in small groups. *Psychological Bulletin*, 63: 384–399.

Tuckman, B. & Jenson, M. (1977). Stages of small-group development revisited. *Group and Organization Studies*, 2(4): 419–427.

Wheelan, S. (2013). *Creating effective teams: A guide for members and leaders*. Thousand Oaks, CA: Sage.

White, J. & Sharma, N. (2012). Podcasting: A technology, not a toy. *Advances in Health Science Education*, 17(4): 601–603.

Wykurz, G. & Kelly, D. (2002). Developing the role of patients as teachers: Literature review. *British Medical Journal*, 325(7368): 818–821.

Yu, T.-C., Wilson, N., Singh, P., Lemanu, D., Hawken, S. & Hill, A. (2011). Medical learners-as-teachers: A systematic review of peer-assisted teaching during medical school. *Advances in Medical Education and Practice*, 2: 157–172.

Zanussi, L., Paget, M., Tworek, J. & McLaughlin, K. (2012). Podcasting in medical education: Can we turn this toy into an effective learning tool? *Advances in Health Science Education*, 17(4): 597–600.

Zarezadeh, Y., Pearson, P. & Dickinson, C. (2009). A model for using reflection to enhance interprofessional education. *International Journal of Education*, 1(1): E12.

CHAPTER 6

Transforming Learning

KEY CONCEPTS
- Changing and transforming practices
- Content
  - Domain knowledge
  - Heuristic strategies
  - Control-support strategies
    - Monitoring
    - Directing
    - Remediation
- Teaching methods to promote clinical learning
  - Modelling
  - Coaching
  - Scaffolding
  - Articulation
  - Reflection
  - Exploration
- Sequencing
- Sociology

INTRODUCTION

Extending educational experiences transforms the learner, the teaching practices and the environment in which learning takes place. In this chapter, we have chosen to use a different approach to assist the teacher facilitate learners' knowledge development and reconstruct their understanding of the practice environment and their capability. The presentation of this chapter reorientates Collins, Brown and Newman's (1989) model of Cognitive Apprenticeship for promoting an ideal learning environment. Their model was originally designed to teach learners to think and problem solve in areas of reading, writing and mathematics. Our interpretation and application of the model acknowledges how teachers can assist learners to develop clinical reasoning and metacognitive skills within the social dimensions and practical contexts of healthcare environments. However, the characteristics can also be extended to assist the learner to become cognisant of themselves, their affective development and the social dimensions to their practice.

An ideal clinical learning environment, to support and encourage learning, aims to promote knowledge development and clinical reasoning alongside health practitioners in professionally situated activities of practice. The framework presented in this chapter assists the teacher's expert understanding of design and teaching methods in the clinical arena. It further recognises the learner's interrelated integration of personal, professional and situated knowledge development as it is reframed by experience.

CHANGING AND TRANSFORMING PRACTICES

Brown and his colleagues (Brown et al., 1989; Collins et al., 1989) describe learning as a 'cognitive apprenticeship'. Brown et al. (1989, p. 237) indicate that a cognitive apprenticeship tries to 'enculturate learners into authentic activity through activity and social interaction'. They identify authentic activities as those framed and defined by the surrounding culture. Culture in this sense is the knowledge and culture of the health profession and all the profession espouses, both explicitly and tacitly. The meaning and purpose of the activities are 'socially constructed through negotiations among present and past members' (p. 34). Therefore, activities and knowledge are accessible to the total practice community, including practitioners, teachers and all types of learners.

The essential function of a cognitive apprenticeship is to engage the learner in higher order cognitive processes to reciprocate externalised knowledge—whether it is technical, scientific, affective or social—between the novice learner and teacher (Brown et al., 1989; Collins et al., 1989). The teacher or experienced practitioner is the custodial facilitator and keeper–transmitter of discipline knowledge. Engagement, then, between teachers and learners not only transmits and carries forward the culture of the profession but will ultimately, over time, allow learners to transform and extend refined practices and notions of the profession (Lave & Wenger, 1991; Lave, 1993, 1997).

Table 6.1 has been adapted to incorporate a range of concepts and outlines strategies and considerations to create an ideal supportive clinical-learning environment for students. The four characteristics to the model are: *content*, *methods*, *sequencing* and *sociology*. Each has a subset of features that provides an intricate web by which to understand not just the creation and evaluation of learning but provides a constructive framework for exploring teaching and learning in practice settings. The processes assist learners to reconstruct their knowledge.

CONTENT

Content refers to the knowledge the expert tacitly uses to develop concepts, facts and procedures necessary to carry out problem solving and activities of professional practice. Content acknowledges the decontextualised facts, definitions and rules that inform

TABLE 6.1	Characteristics of an Ideal Learning Environment (adapted from Collins et al., 1989)	
Content	Domain knowledge	
	Heuristic	
	Control-support strategies	
Methods	Modelling	
	Coaching	Schon (1987)
	Scaffolding and fading	Vygotsky (1978); Spouse (1998)
	Articulation	
	Reflection	Schon (1983, 1987)
	Exploration	
Sequencing	Increasing complexity	
	Increasing diversity	
	Global before local skills	
Sociology	Situated learning	Lave & Wenger (1991)
	Culture of expert practice	
	Intrinsic motivation	
	Making comparisons	
	External environment	

the profession or discipline. Content recognises the connections that empirical knowledge and evidence-based practice have to the total schema of understanding within a healthcare discipline.

As teachers and practice partners provide and support learning opportunities, they also induct learners into the reality of attending and relating to another human being. They alert learners to the dichotomy between textbook and ideal rule-governed learning and expose learners to experiential variations of practice. Often this reveals the subtle way the health professional community's culture is perpetuated.

Content is extended to include *domain knowledge, heuristic strategies,* and *control strategies.*

Domain Knowledge

Domain knowledge is the clearly identified conceptual, factual and procedural subject matter found in textbooks, class lectures, research journals and demonstrations. For health practitioners, this takes into account the learning of health science; of biological and psychosocial sciences and discipline knowledge, and theories of practice. It is only when learners encounter 'real problems' of practice that they can begin to piece together how their tertiary knowledge informs client conditions, management and professional intervention. Therefore, domain knowledge provides a theoretical-background foundation on which to make clinical judgements about individual clients or practice settings.

ACTIVITY 6.1

Complete one task, either (a) *or* (b):

(a) Identify a clinical situation or client to which you are presently assigned. Consider, then write down, the domain knowledge you have drawn on to help inform you and manage the client's treatment or management. How would you use this information when assisting a learner or colleague?

(b) Identify a specific client situation in which both you and the learner are jointly involved. Independently, each draw on your domain knowledge (theoretical knowledge) that you consider has helped inform you of the client's situation or manifestations. Now compare your responses. You can use this information to discuss the similarities and differences, convergence or divergence. It is also an interesting exercise to determine how evidence-based practices (EBPs) have informed you and what gaps in knowledge need to be accessed to assist learning. Reflecting on the exercise, how could you use this information to inform further learning events?

Often learners will want to check their understandings of situations against domain knowledge. They may seek references and reassurances from various sources, and this should be encouraged. Teachers can also use domain resources or other instructional materials to reinforce linkages between theoretical and practical knowledge and extend the learner's comprehension of client situations and clinical activities.

Drawing on the works of Facione (2005) on critical thinking, McAllister et al. (2007) suggest that both visual and verbal resources can assist learners' critical thinking skills. They note that learners need to see how clinical teachers use and manipulate knowledge to inform their clinical practices. The use of supplementary visual or auditory resources also provides information to support verbal explanations.

Such resources can include: visual aids (wall charts, pamphlets), textbooks, clinical procedural material, commercially prepared materials, websites, use of personal digital assistants (PDAs), computer simulations, YouTube©, prepared course material and lecture notes.

ACTIVITY 6.2

Using a client situation, develop a list to determine what extended resources you could use to help learners reinforce and reconstruct their knowledge. Think about what resources are located in your clinical environment. If none is available, identify how you could access further resources to undertake this activity.

Heuristic Strategies

Heuristic strategies are regarded as 'tricks of the trade'. These are often the tacitly acquired, helpful techniques and approaches the expert practitioner uses to solve problems of practice. Heuristic problem solving is situation dependent, because what works in one situation may not work in another. Within the healthcare context, the problems of practice are also client dependent. Therefore, even though each healthcare discipline may use different publicised approaches to problem solving, the expert practitioner often uses other or novel strategies to engage with and adjust to idiosyncratic client presentations (McAllister, 2007; Higgs et al., 2008; Benner et al., 2010). Clinical examples include:

- Effective positioning of clients
- Designing and/or adapting rehabilitation aids
- Involving the client in novel ways: an example may be using a range of distraction techniques (i.e. knowing what and when to use them).

INSIGHT 6.1

All health professions use knowledge acquired from other practitioners. Recall a time that a practitioner used a novel approach to a client problem or used heuristic strategies that caught your attention. In other words, how did they demonstrate a 'trick of the trade'?

Now think about how you have used this information in your own practice. How do you think you could use this information in your future practice or with learners?

How do 'tricks of the trade' sit with your profession's publicised approach to problem solving or dealing with unique client situations?

How could they be incorporated to assist learning?

How can you assist the learner to deconstruct events and practices in order to challenge and change taken-for-granted habits or 'tricks of the trade'?

Another form of heuristic knowledge is the ability to make fine discriminations in practice. An example of this, in many of the health professions, is reliance on forms of touch or palpation. In assisting a learner to develop a 'feel' for certain aspects of touch, the teacher may indicate that 'you can just feel it' or 'you can feel the difference'. This tactile, proprioceptive, kinesthesic-based haptic perception form of learning relies strongly on experience to distinguish the subtle differences in detection of different gradients of 'feel'. These nuances and responses to the client are often difficult to replicate in simulations, but can be rehearsed. However, the particular form of knowing differences can never be represented through domain knowledge but only be nurtured through repetitive and different client presentations.

INSIGHT 6.2

Recall situations where you may use touch, sight, listening or smell to make discriminations in your practice. Consider how you would go about teaching a learner to make clinical judgements about these subtle differences.

As learners develop an increased repertoire of heuristics and strategies for problem solving they are forced to reflect, select and decide which ones to use. Thus, they reconstruct existing knowledge into contextual and discipline knowledge. As we learn and then communicate this knowledge to others, we are transmitting the hidden, sometimes unspoken, almost secretive and often transformed practice knowledge from one generation of practitioners to the next. Unearthing the ways practitioners deal with novel, challenging or complex situations exposes learners to unpublished ways practitioners go about and think in practice. Learners then have the opportunity to scrutinise habits and 'tricks of the trade', deconstructing and reconstructing their use to accept or reject them in their own practices.

Control-Support Strategies

Control strategies are further divided into *monitoring*, *diagnostic* and *remedial strategies*. We have extended control strategies to include *directing* alongside *monitoring*.

Monitoring and Directing

Monitoring and directing by the teacher integrates learner autonomy and client safety. As learners engage in practice, teachers monitor and direct the learner. These activities heighten the learner's awareness of significant aspects of an event and also identify an immediate course of action or a variation to it. In the support strategies of monitoring and directing, the teacher displays concern for the learner by indicating that help is at hand, if required. The teacher acts as a safety net as they monitor learner progress and ensure client safety. Monitoring allows the teacher generally to watch the learner, making sure they are coping with assigned and self-identified activities. The manner displayed by the teacher does not detract from the learner independently undertaking activities of the discipline.

Directing can be defined as verbal nudges or prompts. Teachers use directing by reminding and refocusing the learner on the importance of activities that need to be attended to, or by making suggestions about client management. Directing supports learners' knowledge development through subtle attempts by the teacher, to alert learners to activities that need to be commenced or completed at particular times. Interestingly, as teachers alert learners to these activities, they indirectly help learners to structure their client and professional activities and their time management.

Often the teacher will monitor learners in an extended way, similar to the way they monitor clients. The teacher looks for discriminatory changes in the learner's manner that will inform them of the learner's progress. As the learner evaluates their progress of successful problem resolution, by using published professional criteria, they also effectively detect where and why difficulties arise during their learning process. Therefore, both the teacher and learner diagnose learning deficits (see Table 6.2).

Remediation

Continuing the process, remediation recognises where further learning needs to occur, identifies further activities for resolution, and

TABLE 6.2 Monitoring and Directing Activities
• Displaying concern and interest for the learner
• Acting as a 'safety net'
• Ensuring student copes with assigned activities
• Providing verbal prompts or cues
• Making suggestions
• Observing for change in practice
• Diagnosing learning deficits
• Providing constructive feedback

introduces new knowledge and alternate ways of viewing a problem. Constructive criticism supports learning by providing learners with feedback on their performances. The teacher's actions and verbal cues do not humiliate learners but offer encouragement. The teacher uses constructive criticism with tact and assurance. Chapter 7 discusses feedback in more detail.

Teachers offer learners a significant variety of information on clients and their conditions, organising and making suggestions on how to carry out client activities effectively and efficiently. Through monitoring and directing, teachers help learners to understand the integration of client care, interventions and management to solve problems of and in practice.

INSIGHT 6.3

How do you go about monitoring a learner?

What are you monitoring them for?

What type of directions do you give to learners?

Do these directions include explanations by yourself or the learner?

How do you go about 'diagnosing' a learner?

How do you use this information to assist you and the learner?

METHODS

The second characteristic of an ideal learning environment is method. Method is both a teaching and learning feature. Collins et al. (1989, p. 481) contend that the acquisition and use of teaching methods for problem solving 'should be designed to give learners the opportunity to observe, engage in, and invent or discover expert strategies in context', fostering autonomy and leading to independence. The challenge for teachers and researchers has been to highlight the complex cognitive activities and tacit knowledge, skills and strategies of expert practice, and help make these visible to the learner (Collins et al., 1989; Brown et al., 1989; Schon, 1987; Benner & Sutphen, 2007; Stockhausen, 2006). The characteristics of the six teaching methods of *modelling, coaching, scaffolding and fading, articulation, reflection* and *exploration* (Collins et al., 1989, p. 481) are suggested to promote access to the expert's knowledge.

Modelling

Modelling requires the expert to demonstrate activities (i.e. behavioural modelling) and give a verbal account of their reasoning and decision-making process (cognitive modelling). This allows learners to observe and construct their conceptual model of the indicators, finer points and processes developed through engagement with the activity and for later use in different circumstances (Brown et al., 1989). In their actions and communications, teachers model ways of 'being'. McAllister et al. (2007) also suggest that modelling of this nature can stimulate learners to develop the skill of routinely scrutinising practice and issues surrounding it.

As teachers undertake day-to-day activities, they respond to client situations spontaneously, include learners, and make explanations and rationales for their actions, thus extending learners' ways of 'becoming' health practitioners. Students also develop a construction of their ideal practitioner as they take on board aspects of the expert's practice that they would ideally emulate (Stalmeijer et al., 2009).

> ### ACTIVITY 6.3
>
> **Mapping Decision Making**
>
> Using a current client presentation/situation, generate a decision map. Try to jot down the questions you are asking yourself as you think about the client's situation or problems that require resolution. Ask the learner to do the same. It does not matter at what level the learner is.
>
> Now compare your maps. This will assist you to see how you come to make clinical decisions and your preferred ways of doing things. It will also help you see how the learner is thinking and where they may require assistance to reconsider or expand their knowledge. It also helps the learner to perceive 'how you think'. Sharing and articulating your decision-making processes with the learner helps them to 'get inside your head', to see how the teacher not only makes practical decisions but also resolves problems.

Coaching

Coaching extends modelling as the learner engages with the expert practitioner. Schon (1987) identified three coaching strategies: *follow me*, *joint experimentation* and *hall of mirrors*. These three strategies are not mutually exclusive but traverse and coalesce with one another depending on the learner's ability, the degree of difficulty of a task, the activity and number of times it has been attempted by the learner, and the context in which it occurs.

In 'follow me' coaching, learners suspend judgement, intentions and objectives as the coach tells, demonstrates, is observed, followed and imitated. The coach uses an 'extensive repertoire of media, languages and methods of description' to communicate intentions, discern students' understanding, and question and evaluate interactions. The student attempts to interpret and mimic the coach's actions, investigating constructed meanings to reveal similarities or incongruence with the coach. An essential component of this coaching function is the ability of the coach to 'unpack' whole situations into smaller parts, but also to demonstrate a comprehensive effectiveness between the parts as a whole. This is similar to demonstrating, as outlined in the previous chapter.

Joint-experimentation coaching is initiated through collaborative enquiry by establishing, facilitating (demonstrating and describing) and extending learner-identified goals. The central aspect of this coaching approach lays in the artistry of reciprocity. The student willingly addresses personal learning issues because the coach supports this through joint experimentation. The coach needs to avoid the risk of identifying, answering or resolving learner-initiated issues. Instead, the coach uses their expertise to 'generate a variety of solutions to the problem, leaving the learner free to choose and produce new possibilities for action' (Schon, 1987, p. 296).

The notion of reciprocity is continued in the 'hall of mirrors' coaching function. Here, the student and coach create an atmosphere that explores each other's knowledge development but at the same time acknowledges the uniqueness of each other's knowledge. They practise together; they talk about the enactment and use this to create a model to redesign their practices. As the coach functions in an authentic manner, they model for the student new ways of seeing opportunities to learn. Hall of mirrors replicates students' ideal practitioners and practice to exemplify in their own practice (Schon, 1987, p. 297).

Through the enactment and integration of skills, coaching incorporates situated constructive feedback and helpful hints and reminders, refocusing attention on overlooked aspects of an activity and interactive support. Through the use of genuine regard and positive reinforcement, the learner is offered encouragement and rewarded for their practical attempts. Constructive feedback reinforces positive and appropriate behaviour and tries to extend or apprise learners of the idiosyncrasies in some situations (see Table 6.3).

TABLE 6.3	Elements of Coaching in Clinical Practice

- Modelling practice and behaviours
- Communicating
- Questioning
- Evaluating
- 'Unpacking' wholes into parts
- Establishing, facilitating and extending learners' goals
- Providing constructive feedback
- Giving hints, prompts and reminders

INSIGHT 6.4

Think about the types of responses you make to learners as they attempt new or rehearsed professional activities.

What prompts do you use to remind learners of significant aspects of their practice or client presentations?

In what ways do you offer positive reinforcement and encouragement to learners?

Scaffolding and Fading

Scaffolding determines how much assistance to offer the learner. It structures experiences, building on co-operation, to foster joint activities and learner confidence and independence. Acknowledgement by the teacher and recognition of the learner's level of proficiency is a necessary prerequisite for scaffolding to be successful. Monitoring, directing, modelling and coaching methods help scaffolding.

Initially, the teacher offers assistance through directing practices, reassurances and constructive feedback. As the learner builds a sequential repertoire of skills and confidence, the teacher uses the process of 'fading' or a gradual 'letting go' of the learner, to let them be more independently involved in the practice setting and client management. The learner is also still assured that help is at hand should they require it. Through this process, independence and self-determined practice is fostered. Learners are then required to assume as much of the task on their own, as soon as possible. This also gently nudges the learner to assume responsibility and engage in more intense collaboration with other members of the community of practitioners as they go about the practice of the discipline (see Table 6.4).

INSIGHT 6.5

How do you differentiate between different learners' abilities?

What are your expectations of a first-, second-, third- or fourth-year learner, a postgraduate learner, someone re-entering the workforce or someone new to a specialty of practice? How do you know how much assistance to give each of these learners?

When do you know that a learner has reached a level of ability to undertake activities independently?

How do you foster learner's independence when they have reached a level of proficiency?

What are the boundaries between close supervised practice and safe independent practice?

Does the learner know the difference?

What demonstrates safe initiative?

TABLE 6.4 Scaffolding Clinical Learning

- Providing structure
- Engaging in co-operative activities
- Directing practice
- Providing reassurance
- Offering constructive feedback
- Gradually 'letting go'
- Promoting safe independence

Articulation

Articulation involves actively encouraging learners to articulate how they are thinking by inviting them to think critically. This can be carried out by using provoking questions and having the learner verbalise their thinking aloud as they grapple with a problem situation. Your role is to monitor and critique their responses, recognising gaps in their knowledge or extending their understanding of situations. To assist you, a range of prompt questions is located in Learning Resource 4: Questioning Techniques.

ACTIVITY 6.4

Select an activity you are undertaking with a learner. Invite the learner to 'think aloud' as they assess a client situation. Assist the learner to reconstruct how they are thinking about the client and/or their situation if needed.

Reflection

The fifth method, reflection, enables learners to think back on their observations or experiences and make comparisons as they attempt to make descriptions of the expert, which highlight features of skilful performance. This can be achieved through verbal interactions, either one on one or in groups, or through journals or written assignments. These methods for reflection provide both learner and expert with a replay of events for comparison and growth. Within methods, reflection is identified as a separate entity. However, specific to this book, reflection is integral and not separate from other aspects of method or section. Reflective practices and strategies for reflection help the learner reconstruct their knowledge and are discussed further in the following chapter.

ACTIVITY 6.5

Reflective Observations

Develop a list of significant and salient features of one activity that you commonly undertake.

Or, depending on the level of the learner, focus on just one aspect of the activity that the learner or you have identified as important.

Have a learner observe your practice as you perform (demonstrate) this activity. Using the activity list you developed, make comparisons with the learner about what each of you saw as the activity was being carried out. Discuss with the learner their interpretation of why observations and reflections may converge or differ. Use this information to alert the learner to nuances in the observation and ask how they intend to use this in their future practice.

••

As teachers observe learners or demonstrate professional activities, they see the practice of events unfolding before them. This alerts the teacher to the intricacies of the practice activity. Often the finer components of the skill have been hidden from the teacher's view. As a learner undertakes an activity, the teacher views the activity and reflects in the moment (reflection in action) as if they were the one performing the skill. As such, an internal reflective conversation is provoked with the situation. The triggered reflection in action alerts the teacher to articulate (think aloud) experiential prompts and offer information to the learner on differing aspects of the activity. This exposes learners to the teacher's collective experience of knowing how and knowing why.

Questions the teacher raises with learners demonstrates their thought patterns about an event, revealing the types of normally taken-for-granted questions that a teacher might intrinsically ask of themselves without a learner by their side. In these types of activities, the learner, while not consciously aware of it, is privy to teachers' reflections in action (Stockhausen, 2006).

For learners, this can become frustrating because their rule-governed approach does not enable them to easily see or evaluate discrepancies in practice. Learners do not have the experience of the teacher or practice partner to make distinctions or manipulate variables. As the teacher raises and offers information, the learner becomes aware of smaller components of the activity, grasping fragments of the whole. As the teacher reflects in action, potential for the learner to learn in action is created.

Learning in action is extended as the teacher encourages learners to articulate their knowledge, reasoning or problem-solving processes (Collins et al., 1989). The teacher uses questioning to examine the learner's retention of client information, gauge learner knowledge, invite reflection, probe, and extend the learner's understanding of situations. However, the questions themselves request more than seeking clarification from learners.

INSIGHT 6.6

Often what we do as practitioners has become automatic and just part of our everyday professional repertoire. Stop and think about the knowledge you use in your often taken-for-granted everyday activities, and how you respond to certain situations. How will you recognise moments of expertise and alert and then engage learners in your thought processes?

ACTIVITY 6.6

As you observe the learner in various situations, try to think about what has triggered you to ask a particular question. Think behind the question: what made you ask it? What was present in what you saw, heard, smelt or felt? Use this information to alert the students to how you are thinking about the situation.

Exploration

Exploration encourages the learner to become more autonomous to investigate new and more complex problems independently. Once again, a useful strategy is that, similar to a learning contract where learners can set their own goals, they work towards, evaluate and refine their own progress through self-assessment.

SEQUENCING

The third domain in the learning environment framework is sequencing. Sequencing has three sections: *increasing complexity*, *increasing diversity* and *global before local tasks*, outlined as follows:
- *Increasing complexity*: Repeating the performance of a skill, while gradually increasing its complexity, reinforces a learner's sense of achievement and confidence.
- *Increasing diversity*: Increasing the diversity in which a skill can be used increases the prospect of applying the skill to a variety of conceptual and practical situations. Therefore, learners are more likely to be able to cope when confronted with unfamiliar or novel client circumstances.
- *Global*: Global before local skills provide learners with an overview of the totality of an activity, skill or problem-solving process. It helps the learner see where segments of practice operate within a whole. This can be particularly useful where a skill can take on multiple meanings under different circumstances.

SOCIOLOGY

Sociology is the final dimension of the learning environment framework. Viewed from this perspective, cognitive apprenticeship goes well beyond any individual internal process and locates learning within a community of practitioners in a social context. Along with Collins et al. (1989), we have identified a number of other conditions that extend and embed learning in communities of practice. These are situated learning, the culture of expert practice, intrinsic motivation, making comparisons, and the influence of the external environment. Chapter 3 has already highlighted situated learning, the culture of expert practice and the influence of the external environment. Making comparisons in and of practice is also significantly discussed throughout Chapters 4 to 7.

⌜◉⌝ Snapshot

The complex interplay between the learner and the teacher is enacted as the learner endeavours to reconstruct their discipline knowledge alongside a more competent and experienced practitioner within a clinical environment. The intricate array of learning techniques that the teacher or practice partner can employ throughout this interplay, and the previous phases of clinical learning, contribute to the learner's trajectory on a practice 'experiential ladder'; they build knowledge and provide legitimacy as the learner encounters and interacts with the communities of practitioners and within the practice.

We believe this chapter provides teachers and practice partners with a useful and more meaningful approach than most other texts in considering how they teach and alert learners to nuances of how and what to learn in often unstructured and unpredictable clinical environments. The following chapter, which deals with the Reflection and Reconstructive Learning phase, explores further ways to facilitate learners' understanding of their practice-based experiences.

REFERENCES

Benner, P. & Sutphen, M. (2007). Learning across the professions: The clergy, a case in point. *Journal of Nursing Education*, 46(3): 103–108.

Benner, P., Sutphen, M., Leonard, V. & Day, L. (2010). *Educating nurses: A call for radical transformation*. San Francisco: Jossey-Bass.

Brown J.S., Collins A. & Duguid, P. (1989). Situated cognition and the culture of learning. *Educational Researcher*, 18(1): 32–43.

Collins, A., Brown, J.S. & Newman, S.E. (1989). Cognitive apprenticeship: Teaching the crafts of reading, writing and mathematics. In L.B. Resnick (Ed.), *Knowing, learning and instruction: Essays in honour of Robert Glaser* (pp. 453–494). Hillsdale, NJ: Lawrence Erlbaum Associates.

Facione, P. (2005). Critical thinking: What it is and why it counts. Keynote address presented at the 2nd Ministry of Health International Nursing Conference and 10th Joint Singapore–Malaysian Nursing Conference, Singapore.

Higgs, J. & Titchen, A. (2001). *Professional practice in health, education and the creative arts*. Oxford: Blackwell Science.

Higgs, J., Jones, M.A., Loftus, S. & Christensen, N. (2008). *Clinical reasoning in the health professions* (3rd ed.). Amsterdam, Boston: Butterworth Heinemann/Elsevier.

Lave, J. & Wenger, E. (1991). *Situated learning: Legitimate peripheral participation*. New York: Cambridge University Press.

Lave, J. (1993). Situating learning in communities of practice. In L.B. Resnick, J.M. Levine & S.C. Teasley (Eds), *Perspectives on socially shared cognition* (pp. 17–36). Washington, DC: American Psychological Association.

Lave, J. (1997). The culture of acquisition and the practice of understanding. In D. Kirschner & J. Whitson (Eds). *Situated cognition: Social, semiotic and psychological perspectives* (pp. 17–35). Mahwah, NJ: Lawrence Erlbaum Associates.

McAllister, M. (2007). *Solution focused nursing: Rethinking practice*. London: Macmillan-Palgrave.

McAllister, M., Tower, M. & Walker, R. (2007). Gentle interruptions: Transformative approaches to clinical teaching. *Journal of Nursing Education*, 46(7): 304–312.

Schon, D.A. (1987). *Educating the reflective practitioner*. San Francisco: Jossey-Bass.

Spouse, J. (1998). Scaffolding learner learning in clinical practice. *Nurse Education Today*, 18(4): 259–266.

Stalmeijer, R., Dolmans, D., Wolfhagen, I. & Scherpbier, A. (2009). Cognitive apprenticeship in clinical practice: Can it stimulate learning in the opinion of students? *Advances in Health Science Education*, 14(4): 535–546. Doi: 10.1007/s10459-008-9136-0.

Stockhausen, L. (2006). Métier artistry: Revealing reflection in action in everyday practice. *Nurse Education Today*, 26(1): 54–62.

Vygotsky, L.S. (1978). *Mind in society: The development of higher psychological processes*. Cambridge: Harvard University Press.

CHAPTER 7

Reflection and Reconstructing Learning

KEY CONCEPTS

- Reflective practice
- Helping learners reflect: Strategies for reflection
  - Self-deliberation
  - Journal writing
  - Sharing reflections
  - Debriefing
- Feedback and clinical assessment
  - Providing learner feedback
  - Clinical assessment
    - Formative and summative assessment
    - Self-assessment

INTRODUCTION

This chapter considers how learners and teachers use reflective practice to reconstruct their interpretations of learning and teaching events, and plan for change. The change may be in the form of modified behaviour that fosters interpersonal relationships, personal and professional development, or alternative strategies/interventions in client care. There is a commitment to action as a result of reflection and the learning and teaching experience. Reconstruction of the experience helps to expand views, re-interpret experience and develop strategies for future action. The reflective strategies discussed in this chapter are self-deliberation, journal writing, sharing reflections and debriefing. Through the use of these reflective strategies, both learners and teachers can examine their practices. Reflection, deliberation and reconstructive action generate personal and professional knowledge within the context of where the learning and teaching take place. Understanding reflective practices and using reflective strategies assist learners and teachers to be more discerning in the way they make decisions; it helps them to justify the decisions made and consider their affect on others.

In the course of our professional lives we make countless decisions that affect our clients. Most of these decisions are based on an objective view, but some decisions are based on our personal and professional histories and values, and thus are subjective and intuitive in nature. When our decisions affect other people, objectivity and reasoning become a vital component for the decision. When our decisions, as teachers, affect individual learners, then the criterion for reasoning becomes essential. Feedback to and assessment and evaluation of the learner identifies to the learner and teacher that change has occurred and learning has taken place. The way we communicate our decisions to the learner can assist or delay movement along their trajectory of becoming a reflective and critically thinking professional.

The second part of this chapter provides a commentary on feedback, assessment and evaluation and how these can assist the teacher as they facilitate the learner's development.

REFLECTIVE PRACTICE

Reflection exposes learners to aspects of themselves and their discipline through active learning about the self. The roles within a culture, experiences, professional practices, consequences, amended experiences and guides for future action and experiences are all explored using the processes of reflection. While reflection has the potential to be empowering for learners, it can also be confronting because it exposes learners not only to themselves but to others. It is essential that, in all forms of reflection, the learner feels a sense of security to reveal their emotive responses, their vulnerabilities and, sometimes, their lack of knowledge and safety in experimenting (Johns, 2010).

Attending to learners' emotional needs may take precedence over other aspects of reflection on an experience. If learners are too preoccupied with strong emotional reactions, then learning will take second place. Only through the use of sensitive investigation, conflict resolution skills and the employ of various counselling skills will some learner situations be resolved or diffused.

Exposing students to more than their personal and occasional self-centric thoughts and interpretations of an event requires extending them. All too often the learner's account occludes the client or others involved in the event or their views; the learner imposes and substitutes their own version of events. In reflective narratives, the learner decides on what to include and what to leave out; their accounts determine exposure. The role of the teacher is to broaden the narratives to reveal other possibilities and expose the learner to ways of interrogating what else may be occurring in situations, events and interactions, for not only themselves but for all involved (Taylor, 2010).

For the clinical teacher, reflection does reveal new possibilities for understanding what is occurring as the learner tries to make sense of practical experiences. The processes of reflection provide the learner with the potential to penetrate and explore tacit knowledge, intuitive thought and taken-for-granted assumptions. It offers new insights into what learners really think and feel about the numerous situations they are faced with in the diverse arenas of clinical environments.

HELPING LEARNERS REFLECT: STRATEGIES FOR REFLECTION

Self-deliberation, journaling and debriefing are strategies that facilitate reflection and reconstruction. These strategies allow learners and teachers opportunities to think back on their experiences and highlight significant exemplars and events. Consideration is given to others involved in the learner's practice such as the client, their significant others, peers, the clinical practice partner or teacher, other healthcare professionals, the organisation and the broader community or healthcare and political system. Each of the reflective processes—self-deliberation, journaling and debriefing—may occur at intervals throughout any given day and usually at the end of a clinical day or rotation.

Reflection helps with:

- Making comparisons
- Sorting through relevant and irrelevant data
- Accounting for incongruities within data or experiences
- Extrapolating information
- Using evidence
- Synthesising information; drawing conclusions
- Documenting and informing
- Proposing new courses of action
- Generating research questions for investigation
- Identifying where evidence can be used to analyse or support assumptions, ideas or actions and interactions
- Raising awareness of the historical, socio-cultural and identified economic constraints that operate in social contexts and impact on the self and practice
- Challenging and questioning the validity of one's world view
- Stimulating discourse; acknowledging multiple points of view
- Most importantly, transforming practice (the professions, context, learners and teachers).

Self-Deliberation

Self-deliberation occurs through reflection-on-action and reflection-in-action processes. We often use the self-deliberation process of reflection-on-action when we go over events immediately after an encounter occurs, or at the end of our day as we drift off to sleep, thinking about the people, places and experiences that appeared throughout the day. We think about who said what, what we and others did in particular situations, and we often consider how we would act differently if the situation should occur again (Johns, 2010). This can be recognised as reflection-on-action. Yet there is another form of self-deliberation we often take for granted: this is reflection that occurs as we are carrying out an activity and it is referred to as reflection-in-action (Schon, 1983).

Refection-in-action is a process of an individual internal conversation that is provoked by surprise, variation or a puzzling event within a situation. Similarly, we do not anticipate alternative courses of action or their consequences until some course of action is already underway. This leads to a questioning of our knowledge, an on-the-spot experimentation, and thinking backwards and forwards within the action of the presenting situation (Stockhausen, 2006).

A different perspective of the problem emerges (reframing) during the response to this ongoing action. In redefining (reframing) the problem, event or puzzlement, the learner and clinical teacher can draw on a repertoire of 'examples, images, understanding and actions' (Schon, 1983, p. 66). Indeed, reflection-in-action is when: past experiences are brought to bear on circumstances in situ; previous frames are imposed which highlight certain aspects of phenomena at work in the present situation; and problems are set, the situation reframed, and new or altered problem-solving actions are generated. Usually we refer to this as 'thinking on our feet'.

Journal Writing

Another way reflection occurs is through writing. The activities and insights throughout this book act as prompts for reflection and writing.

Some teachers and learners are familiar with writing their daily thoughts and experiences in a diary. Journal writing extends the concept of a diary and helps the teacher and learner make sense of experiences.

Journaling is a form of writing to learn; it is a way of thinking and learning that promotes critical thought. Writing provides a personal retrospective and an interpretive questioning and exploration of the concepts learned and applied to the realities of the clinical environment. Johns (2010) also contends that journaling gives voice to self-expression to highlight satisfaction or pride in decisions and outcomes that may be otherwise unacknowledged.

Writing journal entries enhances the learner's ability to move progressively to higher levels of abstraction, to conceptualise, to think; but more importantly it can be a dialogue with oneself that helps understand practice and beliefs (Schon, 1987; Hendrix et al., 2012). Writing to learn is speculative. It allows the learner the freedom and safety to express feelings, experiment, to order and represent their own learning and think about certain issues and events confronting them in their daily practice.

Within the clinical context, journaling allows the learner to write how they think and feel. Journal writing generates personal and professional practice questions and allows for free expression. In this sense, a journal becomes an internal conversation providing the learner (or teacher) with a personal map of issues relevant only to the writer. Valuing the journal by all, as a learning device, is paramount.

Writing can be used to:

- State an opinion
- Examine an idea
- Express feelings
- Share experiences
- Clarify thoughts
- Record impressions
- Examine self-thoughts
- Capture and describe encounters, situations or events
- Manipulate and make links between ideas
- Analyse thoughts, actions, events and interactions.

When to Write

Journal entries can be made close to the time of the experience or to reflect back over a day or number of days. Reference is made to the significance of writing close to, immediately after, or as close as possible to the initial event. This helps capture the original experience before it becomes distorted by new events that may obscure or alter the reflection.

However, it should be noted that writing should be encouraged when it feels right to do so, by either the learner or teacher. This could occur immediately after an event, during debriefing sessions or away from the site in a more relaxed atmosphere. The key is, if it feels like it is the right time to make a journal entry, then do so (Johns, 2010).

Personal Journal Writing

Make it personal. After all, it is personal thoughts, feelings, responses and interpretations that are being recorded (see Box 7.1).

In today's electronic society, personal digital assistants (PDAs) and computers are increasingly being used. These too can also be personalised and used to track clinical practice development. Technologies such as weblogs (blogs) can be useful as an interactive reflective journal. Blogs allow users to make entries publicly or privately available for comment and discussion by others (Miyazoe & Anderson, 2010). Reading and examining one's own and others'

BOX 7.1 Personalising a Journal

In the past I covered my journal in paper that had my name stamped all over it, or attached photos of my family on the front cover. I was creative, adventurous; it was my own space! I also included jokes, diagrams, poetry, comic strips, newspaper articles and doodles.
I reflected on all of these additions, considering why I thought they were relevant to my journal at that time, and the connections and meanings to my personal life and professional practice. Essentially, my journal said something about me; it depicted my growth as a person and professional.

writing allows for interrogation to take place. Teachers can help learners engage in the task of journaling.

Getting Started: Prompts for Writing

Sometimes learners struggle to write and motivators, prompts or key questions can assist both the learner and clinical teacher to get underway. Table 7.1 adapts a number of authors' ideas that act as prompts to writing (Holly, 1987; Lincoln et al., 1997; Johns, 2010).

TABLE 7.1 Prompts for Reflection and Writing Journals

- I was surprised by ...
- I was anxious when ...
- The most important thing I noticed was ...
- What went well for you as you performed the ...
- What was going on when ...
- What were you thinking when ...
- Why did you feel that way?
- Tell me, or us, why you responded in that way?
- What did you consider you accomplished during ...
- What else could you have done at that point?
- If you had done that, what do you think the consequences would have been?
- Tell me, or us, about the time when ...
- What do you think the client wanted to say and why?
- What do you think you would be more aware of now?
- What threat is involved for me if I ...
- Why did the incident cause disquiet and challenge assumptions, beliefs or attitudes?
- How do your reflective journal writings demonstrate movement towards the achievement of your clinical objectives?
- What themes seem to be reoccurring as you write?
- What do your journal writings say about you as a learner or a beginning practitioner?
- How will this learning prepare you for your future practice?

ACTIVITY 7.1

Reflect on your own experiences as a teacher. What can you add to the list in Table 7.1?

Develop a list of prompt questions to assist learners on their quest towards becoming reflective and valuing journal writing. By doing this, the clinical teacher can help the learner develop curiosity, which fosters a deeper level of learning and habits to reflect critically.

Reflect on how journaling can also be a useful tool for the clinical teacher to examine contextual learning, teaching and professional development.

. . . .

Types of Writing

Once learners see the true value of journaling, their individual writing and reflections will vary considerably. To learn through experiences, reflective writing needs to be thoughtful, deliberate and considerate. The learner will and should be encouraged to use a variety of writing styles to extend their learning. Several types of writing styles have been suggested, such as 'journalistic, analytic, ethnographic, creative therapeutic and introspective' styles (Holly, 1987, p. 11).

Journalistic writing is descriptive and interpretative and takes an outsider-observer view of an event. An analytical style of writing examines parts or elements of a topic under study. Thinking, reasoning and relationships among the parts are highlighted. Observations and descriptions of people in specific social and cultural contexts are viewed as ethnographic writing. The writer becomes an observer, making field notes of events and people.

Creative-therapeutic writing, on the other hand, is free flowing, sometimes poetic and spontaneous in nature. This form of writing encourages the creator to reveal the inner self and feelings generated as a consequence of the lived experience. Some people write poetry, draw, or even use photography to express themselves. Introspective writing is perhaps the most confronting and perplexing form of writing. It involves surfacing taken-for-granted behaviours, attitudes, beliefs and values, and examining and transforming them to a conscious level in order to lead to new perspectives and changed practices (Mezirow, 2009).

Encouraging reflection involves writing using a combination of all styles.

Tips on Helping Learners with Their Journals

Some tips the teacher can encourage the learner with are as follows:

- A journal is a personal document. There is no right or wrong way. Keep it personal. It is an extension of yourself. You should say what you feel and think. It also gives you permission to safely experiment with your thinking and your writing.
- Be frank and honest in your writings. Write it as it is, not as you would like it to be, or as you think it should be or that others expect it to be.
- Have a positive approach to your journal. Treat it as a close friend.
- Be aggressive about your journal. Write, write, and write. Let it flow uncensored.
- Use the journal to express yourself: write, use diagrams, pictures, poetry or hyperlinks.
- The journal is a workbook, a think book. Develop an enquiring and questioning approach to what you think and write.
- Work through entries a number of times. Highlight important entries. Use different colours, circling or underlining, to emphasise points. It is important to go back, re-read entries and to reconsider them. You might want to leave a space at the end of an entry for later reflection.
- Be spontaneous. Use your own words. Do not be concerned with the mechanics of academic writing.
- Persevere with it; stick at it.
- If applicable, negotiate confidentiality and who has access to your journal and why.

As a communicative device, journal writing says something about the ways learners view themselves and their practice world.

Sharing Reflections

Encouraging the learner to share journal comments with a trusted colleague or teacher can further enhance understanding of situations. Viewed through different eyes, a friend or teacher may be able to see issues within the writing that the learner might not yet have explored or connected with. Sharing with colleagues can also foster open collegial relationships, offering different versions of the same practice encounter, thus extending the learner and peers' understanding of the event. As learners share their stories they enter into the experiences of one another. They develop a shared sense of excitement, anxiety, relief, or views on how a client felt or responded to care (Stockhausen, 2008).

An important point to remember when learners share reflections is maintaining confidentiality. Teachers must understand all forms of communication that both they and the learners use. Reminding the learner about their ethical and professional-standards responsibilities is paramount. This is particularly relevant when it comes to social networking and mobile communication (Cain, 2008). Safety for the learner is also important. If the learner is sharing their writing with a colleague(s) or the teacher, then trust and discretion is essential. The learner does not want their innermost thoughts broadcast to everyone or the whole organisation, for this could be harmful.

Debriefing

Debriefing can be viewed as another type of reflective conversation. We use informal debriefing such as our conversations about our work, events, clients and the people we come in contact with in our day-to-day life. These conversations often occur at meal breaks or with family, friends and colleagues in relaxed settings. We essentially use group conversations to reflect on our experiences.

Historically, this ad hoc approach diffused many reactions to the unpredictable nature of healthcare work. Although these informal debriefings had the potential to be beneficial, they were random in their resolution or re-orientations for future action. Today, debriefing is a formalised teaching and learning strategy in many education programs.

Debriefing is viewed as a process whereby we reflect on, discuss and work through ideas, issues, feelings or concerns that have been generated by our involvement in an experience (Mackenzie, 2002). Through conversation with others, debriefing allows individuals to share their points of view, name and process emotional reactions, analyse the social and clinical aspects of the situation (Rudolph et al., 2008), grapple with inconsistencies and differences, view similarities, and come to see an experience as a catalyst for future learning and action.

Consulting the literature, debriefing is viewed from a number of perspectives. First of all, there is an inordinate amount of literature that stems from critical-incident stress debriefing used in psychology. While some health practitioners may benefit from this form of debriefing following stressful events, it does not seem appropriate that all educational experiences should be approached in the same way. Nonetheless, some strategies derived from this viewpoint provide useful techniques that can be incorporated into debriefings in confronting situations in the healthcare field, and should not be dismissed (Fink, 2003).

If this is an area you are interested in then consulting the literature may provide you with some strategies for conducting educative debriefing sessions or information sessions for staff development. However, one must keep in mind the educational focus of debriefing and the role of the teacher is not that of a counsellor.

The second form of debriefing stems from an educational perspective. Here debriefing is viewed in the context of experiential and transformational learning, where reflective discourse is seen as a pivotal educational process vital to assist learners to learn and transform themselves from their experiences (Mezirow, 2009). The essential focus of an educative debriefing is that, by allocating time for learners to reflect on and/or share experiences through one-on-one or group conversations, experiences can be reframed to lead to a different perspective for future practice (Zigmont et al., 2011; Cant

& Cooper, 2011) Not every aspect of an event, day or period of time is suitable to be discussed. It is generally recognised that a designated period of time should be set aside for debriefing at the end of each clinical day or rotation, or following a personal experience of significance (Williams & Watson, 2004).

Key Points

The key points for conducting an educational debrief are to:
- Establish the purpose and parameters of the debriefing with the individual or group.
- Foster a climate of trust so the learner feels safe with the teacher and or their peers to discuss all aspects of the encounters they have had.
- Always open a debriefing session with a positive comment.
- Allow the learner to lead the discussion; after all, it is their own experience.
- Provide space for active listening and reflecting while not suppressing participation.
- Deal with emotive aspects first. Let students vent frustrations in a positive way. Learners who may have had a negative or embarrassing encounter may suppress or have a distorted view of the event. Guide students' thoughts to challenge their own views of events to see why some situations occur.
- Invite learners to recall and share their description of events. Call upon quieter learners to comment on other learners' responses.
- Help learners focus on key elements of the story; use reflective questioning.
- Invite discussion from group participants so all students have a voice.
- Provoke inquisitiveness.
- Tease out situations objectively, ethically and non-judgementally.
- Challenge learners' knowledge bases by inviting them to make comparisons between their theoretical understandings and their recent practical observations and experiences.

- Provide key topics to trigger or focus some debriefings. Connect this to the learners' experiences.
- Allow for appropriate silences to prompt further reflection and ponder responses.
- Provide positive feedback where appropriate.
- Focus learners on what has changed for them as a consequence of being involved and reflecting on their clinical experiences, either individually or collectively.
- Provide guidance and allow learners to decide on a new course of action and goals as a consequence of the experience and debriefing exercise.

Individual Debriefing

One-on-one debriefing is usually conducted directly following a clinical encounter. It allows the learner to appraise and reflect immediately on their performance. The learner is encouraged to recall aspects of significance. It is important to prompt the learner to seek first the positive aspects of the event. All too often the learner is eager to identify what they perceive they did wrong. This should be discouraged so the learner can also see they have achieved something and have a sense of accomplishment. The role of the teacher is to provide constructive feedback and ask non-directive questions. This assists the learner to make connections and think about how they will use this experience to inform future practices.

Group Debriefing

In group debriefings, each learner is given the opportunity to relate to the rest of the group an important aspect of their experience. The debriefing therefore becomes a time for learners to share feelings, thoughts and perceptions with one another and to construct a shared understanding of the issue at hand. It allows learners to explore the meaning of their experience from multiple perspectives. Learners have the opportunity to exchange ideas, expand views, draw conclusions and make comparisons from their experiences (Levett-Jones

& Lapkin, 2012). From an interprofessional perspective, Zarezadeh et al. (2009) consider that this process helps learners understand professional roles, reduce prejudices, and foster respect and appreciation. As learners share one another's achievements, experiences, challenges and embarrassments, they enter one another's worlds and opportunities for vicarious learning can take place.

Reference to actual journal entries during the debriefing session can motivate learners to ensure their entries are thorough, honest and meaningful. In this sense, journal writing as a reflective tool fosters critical openness and the development of open collegial relationships with peers, the practice partner or teacher. All participants share their educational experiences.

As a consequence of planned reflection, learners arrive at a deeper and more meaningful understanding of disciplinary practices. Reflective debriefing sets the scene to examine complexities, differences and subtleties often not found in textbooks but which are learned, or made explicit, as a direct result of being emerged in the experience.

Teacher's Role in Debriefing

Because participation is essential to group debriefing, the principal role of the teacher is to be proficient in group-process facilitation. Your approach to facilitation will invariably change according to the group of learners. However, with any group activity, creating the appropriate learning environment is a key consideration.

The teacher is required to develop and maintain a level of trust in a non-judgemental environment where learners feel confident and safe to engage in meaningful conversations and will listen actively to the stories of their peers, constructing meaning for all involved. A permissive atmosphere encourages freedom of exploration and freedom of expression without reprisal.

Experience alerts the teacher to aspects of encounters and events that might not have been considered by the student or group. The teacher poses problems and questions to seek validation and information, explore alternatives, re-focus learners on important aspects of the topic under discussion, clarify points of view, and highlight inconsistencies (Mayville, 2011). In debriefing it is not primarily the role of the teacher to answer questions posed but to instigate extending learners beyond their initial ideas and responses.

Reflection can be initiated at anytime on a one-on-one basis between a learner and clinical practice partner, peer or other staff. It is particularly important to provide reflective time for constructive feedback to learners following some aspect of their practice development. This may be a psychomotor skill, interpersonal interaction or professional enquiry, for example. Later, during group debriefing, learners have opportunities to share personal reflections from their previous one-to-one reflection or share extracts from their journals.

In the group setting, a set of negotiated, mutual goals can be developed as a consequence of reflections on experiences, journal entries and discussions during debriefings. It is the participants of the educative experience who decide if reflections develop into action (Stockhausen, 1994). It is essential that the actions decided upon are not imposed on learners, because it is the learner's engagement with all aspects of the educative experience that culminates in meaning and learning and the exposure of future actions.

Either as individuals or as a group, and as a consequence of experience and reflection, new and changed understandings of oneself, others and practice are produced. Goals are recreated as a direct result of practice. The intention is to modify or develop new goals that can be enacted during the next educational experience. It is imperative that a commitment to action as a consequence of the experiences and reflections is realised (Johns, 2010). Action without reflection can lead to uninformed, unintentional behaviour. Reflection prior and subsequent to action can ensure personal and mutual goals are carried forward to the next situation.

ACTIVITY 7.2

When facilitating debriefing sessions, identify when you undertake the following roles and what you do while in them that promotes active learner engagement and student learning:

• Manager

• Adjudicator

• Mediator

• Motivator

• Co-contributor

• Generator of feedback

• Change agent/catalyst.

Reflection in Review

In review, self-deliberation, journal writing and debriefing provide avenues for learners to develop reflectivity by:
  • Safely experimenting with and refining their own written and oral expression
  • Developing reflection as a lifelong skill
  • Thinking about individual problems
  • Increasing confidence in interpersonal relations
  • Integrating ways of knowing (empirical, practical, aesthetic, ethical and moral)
  • Safely challenging accepted ways of doing things
  • Having better peer and teacher understandings
  • Becoming more fluent in creative expression
  • Becoming confident that opinions are valued
  • Manipulating and making links between ideas
  • Making knowledge of self and the world more meaningful
  • Exposing ideological perspectives

- Raising awareness of historical, economic, political and socio-cultural influences
- Expanding an understanding of the roles and responsibilities of the healthcare team and organisation.

Reflection and reflective strategies can be used to help both the learner and teacher make sense of educational experiences. Practical knowledge development is generated through engagement with the world by deliberating and reflecting upon it. Knowledge cannot be given, it must be constructed, and so understanding is an internal process of creating knowledge through the ways we think about the world. When you reflect in terms of your own reactions and responses, you discover that your ideas are potentially as powerful as any others'.

Reflection exposes practitioners, whether novice or experienced, to aspects of themselves and their discipline by actively involving learning about the self. Roles within a culture, experiences, consequences, amended experiences and the guides for future action are all explored using the processes of reflection.

Reflection does reveal new possibilities for us to understand what is occurring in our educational experiences. The processes of reflection provide us with the potential to penetrate and explore our tacit knowledge and intuitive thought. It offers new insights into what we really think and feel about the numerous situations we are faced with in different educational situations.

In an environment of trust, learners and the teacher can both expose their actions, thoughts and feelings; they can hold them up for examination, recreate them and then transform them. In so doing, learners are likely to question and challenge their preconceived assumptions about professional practice.

Schon (1983) asserts that, through reflective practice, learners develop a critical understanding of the repetitive experiences of a specialised practice and can make new sense of any situations of uncertainty or uniqueness they experience. These experiences lie within a lived context, which is connected to the learners' reality within that context.

FEEDBACK AND CLINICAL ASSESSMENT

Providing Learner Feedback

Effective feedback is continuous and constructive. You will note that reinforcing professional behaviours and providing correctional support is ongoing throughout the learner's clinical experience. This has been highlighted in previous chapters. Nicol and Macfarlane-Dick (2006, p. 205) provide seven principles of sound feedback practice, in that it:

1. Helps clarify what good performance is (goals, criteria, expected standards)
2. Facilitates the development of self-assessment (reflection) in learning
3. Delivers high quality information to students about their learning
4. Encourages teacher and peer dialogue around learning
5. Encourages positive motivational beliefs and self-esteem
6. Provides opportunities to close the gap between current and desired performance
7. Provides information to teachers that can shape teaching.

The role of the teacher in giving feedback to the learner is to provide a supportive and non-judgemental atmosphere to stimulate learner recall (or reflect on experiences), provide reinforcement, highlight strengths and recognise difficulties the learner may be experiencing. Constructive feedback reinforces to the learner appropriate behaviours, affirms achievements and assists the underperforming learner to modify their performance within realistic timeframes. Communicating this feedback in a sensitive manner and in a supportive context aids in providing constructive criticism to the learner so they can gauge their progress and make adjustments.

Sometimes feedback is used as a reinforcer and can occur in a matter of seconds. An example of this is the way a simple 'that was great' directed at a learner's performance attempt can boost their self-esteem and give them confidence to progress. Pursed lips, disparaging remarks, head shakes, not commenting or commenting under one's breath can also just as easily discourage or destroy a learner's self-esteem. Therefore, the delivery of the feedback is important. For the teacher this can sometimes be frustrating and difficult, particularly where a learner's behaviour has been inappropriate or jeopardised client safety. Being aware of your own reactions is imperative. It is important not to release your anger or frustration on the learner. Ensure you have time to reflect and disperse your reactions to develop a meaningful response. Belittling a learner in front of others can harm their self-esteem and confidence.

Your feedback should be confidential, addressed only to the learner, away from the client, not in front of others, and removed from the situation. In the busy clinical environment this may require planning. Ensure feedback is provided in a quiet area away from distractions or interruptions, other students and health professionals (Hill, 2007).

Establishing the purpose of the feedback provides a focus on individual learning requirements. In offering feedback, the teacher first invites the learner to reflect on the event or interaction. This demonstrates that the learner's responses and reactions to the experience are valued by the teacher. Acknowledging and building upon the learner's ideas fosters open communication. It provides an avenue to be sensitive to the learner's intent and responsive to reinforce positive outcomes while highlighting areas for improvement.

Be alert to the learner being open to receive feedback and prepared to consider your comments, which may be different from their own perceptions. Correctional feedback is often the most difficult for the teacher to deliver. Sometimes the learner is unaware of their behaviour and, when confronted with negative feedback, is shocked and dismayed. For some learners, it can be demoralising while others will see it as an opportunity to improve or change their practices. For feedback to be meaningful it needs to be specific and given immediately or as close to the event as possible. Delayed or general feedback has little significance.

Specific feedback requires that it is related to the precise situation or interaction under discussion. As the provider of the feedback you need to state as accurately as possible your reactions, both positive and/or negative, and your interpretation of the event. Verify your responses by giving examples, by explaining consequences, and use this information as it relates to professional behaviours. Such a process allows the learner to view their actions from another perspective and use this to improve behaviours. Raising personal or personality matters rather than performance issues can leave the learner feeling vulnerable. It is important that the teacher focuses on the situation, issue or behaviour and not the learner personally. This is one of a number of hazards to avoid when providing feedback.

Not using second-hand information, based on hearsay, ensures the feedback is accurate. You are providing feedback to the learner, not an array of complaints from others. Avoid the use of an extensive list of deferred negative and vague comments, because these can often be overwhelming for the learner to comprehend. They can become preoccupied with the perceived affront rather than on the actual content being discussed. Often the learner becomes defensive, may cry or become angry. In these situations, provide space for the learner to reflect. Allow time for silence so the learner has time to think. Listen to their responses, and seek clarification by confirming your understanding of the learner's remarks. Using combinations of paraphrasing and perception-checking, you can garner where discrepancies exist between the learner's account of events and your own, and identify misunderstandings and misinterpretations.

When the learner is ready, ask them how they think they will be able to use the feedback to make adjustments. Allowing the learner to think through solutions fosters their self-awareness and provides them with an avenue to work constructively through difficulties or challenges. Suggesting practical and realistic ways in which the learner will be able to move forward can be useful. In showing genuine regard for the learner, you demonstrate that correctional feedback can be used for professional growth.

In some situations it is necessary to provide feedback to the learner's university or immediate supervisor. In these cases it is imperative that your judgements are supported by specific written examples of the learner's inability to conduct themselves at an agreed, negotiated or appropriate level or within safe requirements. Table 7.2 summarises suggestions for feedback in clinical settings.

Verbal and Non-Verbal Reinforcers

Verbal and non-verbal reinforcers need to vary in type, amount and intensity. Commendations, praise, suggestions for extending the learner's initial ideas or challenging the learner's ideas can foster self-esteem and motivation. Correctional starters are sometime difficult but can be expressed in such a manner that highlight to the learner that help is at hand. Table 7.3 provides some examples of reinforcers.

ACTIVITY 7.3

Consult your colleagues and further literature to add to the lists in Table 7.3.

Feedback, both verbal and non-verbal, can be used at regular intervals to assist both the teacher and learner to make judgements about progress. Formal feedback sessions at a midpoint during the practical experience are useful for the teacher and learner to check progress is being made—that clinical objectives identified in the learning contract are being achieved—and to identify the strengths and areas for

---

TABLE 7.2 Corrective Feedback in the Clinical Setting: Key Points

- Make it constructive, supportive and objective
- Ensure privacy
- Offer guidance for future development and promote learning
- Seek learners' perceptions
- Be aware of your own and the learner's feelings
- Focus on the situation, issue or behaviour and not the learner themselves
- Avoid use of second-hand information and hearsay

improvement or change. Midpoint feedback also provides time for the learner to rectify behaviours and knowledge deficits to achieve positive learning outcomes. Feedback also becomes a conduit for assessment and evaluation.

••

TABLE 7.3	Examples of Reinforcers
Non-verbal	• Smiles • Head nods • Eye contact • Attentive listening • Positive written comments
Verbal	*Reaffirming* • You performed that … proficiently • I liked the way you … • The way you drew the client into discussion shows you have successfully … • You certainly seem to have grasped the importance of … by the way you … • I was impressed when you …
	Correctional • Do you have any concerns? • Have you considered …? • I have some concerns regarding … • I was concerned when you … • How might you do … differently next time? • [*Name*], tell me what your reactions or interpretations of the event were.
	Novel reinforcers • Suggest the learner presents their ideas to others (peers, other professionals) • Suggest the student adds the feedback to their portfolio or reflections

INSIGHT 7.1

Consider your own teaching and the feedback you provide to learners.

Do you identify specific strengths and weaknesses to the learner and offer precise feedback to improve performance? From your reading, what other strategies could you incorporate?

Clinical Assessment

Assessment begins early in the learner–teacher relationship. It depends on the entry level of the learner, the assistance required by the learner, and the attainment or otherwise of the learner's identified learning objectives and their relationship to the formal curriculum aims for the clinical experience.

Formative and Summative Assessment

Undertaking student assessment can be one of the most difficult roles of being a teacher. The observations we make of the learner throughout their entire experience provide information for assessment.

There are two different types of assessment: formative and summative. Formative assessment is often done informally throughout the learning or clinical experience. Most often this is not a written assessment, but is provided via ongoing verbal feedback for the learner on their performance. Summative assessment is usually a more formal assessment carried out at the end of a unit of study or placement experience. Here the teacher is often required to make a judgement, which, in a clinical context, may be either a pass or fail, satisfactory or unsatisfactory. However, the key function of assessment is to provide the learner with formal feedback to facilitate professional development (Hays, 2008).

In the clinical setting, summative assessment is largely related to clinical competence. Many disciplines have professional competency standards that form the basis of the clinical assessment tool. These are designed to ensure the assessment is valid (it measures what it sets out to measure), reliable (the consistency by which it measures what it needs to) and objective (based on actual observation). That being said, there is often an element of subjectivity that influences the assessment—we are, after all, only human! However, it is important to be aware of your own potential subjectivity in assessing students. In one example, Belinsky and Tataronis (2007) found that clinical teachers in radiation therapy tended to use their own past experiences of clinical assessment with their students. If they had positive experiences, teachers tended to be positive to students in assessments, and vice versa. When undertaking objective assessments, there are a number of aspects to consider, including:

- *Distinguishing fact from opinion*: You can do this by looking for the authority and assumptions on which statements are made.
- *Distinguishing observations from inferences*: This can be done by systematically distinguishing one from the other.
- *Identifying errors*: Look for the possibility of errors in measurement, logical fallacies in arguments and invalid conclusions being drawn.
- *Evaluating the worth of ideas*: Critically examine the adequacy of the data, the validity of conclusions and the value of specific claims being made.

INSIGHT 7.2

Access and review the professional standards or competencies relating to your discipline. How do you work towards ensuring that learners are able to achieve these in your clinical setting?

Another important aspect to consider in assessment relates to the ethical component. All teachers possess a number of different accountabilities in the assessment process. These include accountabilities to the learner, clients, the profession, and the university. Hence there is a moral obligation to assess fairly and objectively.

INSIGHT 7.3

Consider your own approach to assessment. In what ways do you ensure that your assessment of the learner is valid, just and ethical?

What Should Be Assessed?

One of the important considerations in undertaking assessment involves determining exactly what components will be assessed. Usually there are formal assessment requirements from the academic centre that need to be achieved. Most often these are stated in specific learning objectives for the learning experience and may include some demonstration that knowledge, technical ability and professional attitudes are developing and are being achieved. The learner may be required to show objective evidence that they have engaged in a sufficient number and range of clinical situations for you to be confident of their goal achievement and progress towards competence. This may be particularly pertinent where you are required to assess a learner's reflective practice. The second section of Chapter 4 discusses the development of learning outcomes in detail. Approaches to their assessment may be:

- *Negotiated or formal*: The learner may be required to negotiate learning outcomes with you on commencement of a clinical placement and/or have formal learning outcomes to be achieved.
- *Negotiated in a learning contract*: The learner may be required to develop a learning contract with you to determine appropriate learning outcomes for the experience.
- *Presented in a clinical portfolio*: The learner may be required to collect evidence of particular learning episodes to contribute to a clinical learning portfolio. This may include reflections on care episodes, experiences in the interprofessional team, or evidence of clinical skills performed (Stuart, 2004).

How Should It Be Assessed?

Not all assessments will be done in the same way. Depending on the particular requirement, an assessment may be done through:

- Negotiation or formal review of learning objectives
- Observation
- Demonstration
- Questioning
- Documentation
- Using set criteria or rating scales
- Repetition.

Why Should It Be Assessed?

Assessment is undertaken to meet a range of requirements. These include:

- Providing a record of evidence and integration of achievement of learning outcomes identified in the formal curriculum and the objectives of the clinical experience, both formal and those identified by the learner
- Helping to build a progressive profile of the learner's achievements
- Motivating the learner to develop further
- Monitoring progress towards professional standards
- Building learner confidence
- Providing guidance for future development.

Who Should Carry Out the Clinical Assessment?

In most cases, the clinical teacher will be the person responsible for a student's clinical assessment. However, depending on the type of placement, the assessor may be a clinician or other health professional. This person may or may not be one appointed by a university, or have a particular understanding of the individual university requirements. In some cases, the assessor may even be a student peer. In identifying suitable clinical assessors, it is important for the person to possess:

- Clinical competence (may not always be the case with peers)
- Sound knowledge of what is being assessed (subject matter)
- Appropriate interpersonal and communication skills to conduct assessments.

INSIGHT 7.4

Consider your experiences as an assessor in the clinical setting. Select one particular challenge you faced in that role. Did you handle the situation well? What could you have done differently?

Self-Assessment

This final section describes self-assessment as it relates to reflection. Learner self-assessment requires the learner to identify and make judgements about their own strengths and weaknesses, movement towards and success in the achievement of personal and professional goals in their learning contract and academic curriculum. Self-assessment is one means by which we, as professionals, undertake reflective practice and work to develop our professional expertise. The process requires honesty and integrity as well as the ability to see different ways of working that may be more effective. All teachers play an important role in promoting learners' abilities in ongoing self-assessment and reflection. Students should be encouraged to undertake self-reflection throughout the learning experience, as well as at the end. It is useful to include a self-assessment format in the clinical portfolio (Stuart, 2004) as evidence of ongoing professional development.

INSIGHT 7.5

Consider your day-to-day work with learners. How do you assist them to develop habits of routinely assessing their own work? Using what you have learnt in this chapter, are there other ways you can promote learner self-assessment?

⟨◎⟩ SNAPSHOT

The reflective phase provides the learner and teacher with opportunities to explore practice and plan for change. Such change may involve alternative strategies or interventions in client care, or changes in behaviour that foster interpersonal relationships or personal and professional development. This chapter explores a range of strategies for promoting learner reflection such as journaling and debriefing. The second half of the chapter examines the roles of feedback and assessment to enhance both learner reflection and professional role development.

REFERENCES

Belinsky, S.B. & Tataronis, G.R. (2007). Past experiences of the clinical instructor and current attitudes toward evaluation of students. *Journal of Allied Health*, 36(1): 11–16.

Cain, J. (2008). Online social networking issues within academia and pharmacy education. *American Journal of Pharmaceutical Education*, 72(1): 1–7.

Cant, R. & Cooper, S. (2011). The benefits of debriefing as formative feedback in nurse education. *Australian Journal of Advanced Nursing*, 29(1): 37–47.

Fink, N.R. (2003). Deaths. *Canadian Medical Association Journal*, 169(8): 887.

Hays, R. (2008). Assessment in medical education: Roles for clinical teachers. *The Clinical Teacher*, 5: 23–27.

Hendrix, T., O'Malley, M., Sullivan, C. & Carmon, B. (2012). Nursing student perceptions of reflective journaling: A conjoint value analysis. *ISRN Nursing (International Scholarly Research Network)*, volume 2012, article ID 317372, 8 pages, doi: 10.5402/2012/317372.

Hill, F. (2007). Feedback to enhance students learning: Facilitating interactive feedback on clinical skills. *International Journal of Clinical Skills*, 1(1): 21–24.

Holly, M.L. (1987). *Keeping a personal–professional journal*. Geelong, Vic.: Deakin University Press.

Johns, C. (2010). *Guided reflection: A narrative approach to advancing professional practice*. West Sussex, UK: Blackwell Publishing.

Levett-Jones, T. & Lapkin, S. (2012). The effectiveness of debriefing in simulation-based learning for health professionals: A systematic review. *Joanna Briggs Library of Systematic Review Protocols*, 10: 3295–3337.

Lincoln, M., Stockhausen, L. & Maloney, D. (1997). Learning processes in clinical education. In L. McAllister, M. Lincoln, S. McLeod & D. Maloney (Eds), *Facilitating learning in clinical settings* (pp. 99–129). Cheltenham, UK: Stanley Thornes.

Mackenzie, L. (2002). Briefing and debriefing of student fieldwork experiences: Exploring concerns and reflecting on practice. *Australian Occupational Therapy Journal*, 49(2): 82–92.

Mayville, M. (2011). Debriefing the essential steps in simulation. *Newborn and Infant Nursing Reviews*, 11(1): 35–39.

Mezirow, J. (2009). Transformative learning theory. In J. Mezirow, E. Taylor and Associates (Eds), *Transformative learning in practice: Insights from community, workplace and higher education*. San Francisco, CA: Jossey-Bass.

Miyazoe, T. & Anderson, T. (2010). Learning outcomes and students' perceptions of online writing: Simultaneous implementation of a forum, blog, and wiki in an EFL blended learning setting. *System*, 38: 185–199e.

Nicol, D.J. & Macfarlane-Dick, D. (2006). Formative assessment and self-regulated learning: A model and seven principles of good feedback practice. *Studies in Higher Education*, 31(2): 199–218.

Rudolph, J., Simon, R., Raemer, D. & Eppich, W. (2008). Debriefing as formative assessment: Closing performance gaps in medical education. *Academic Emergency Medicine*, 15(11): 1010–1016.

Schon, D.A. (1983). *The reflective practitioner*. London: Temple Smith.

Schon, D.A. (1987). *Educating the reflective practitioner*. San Francisco, CA: Jossey-Bass Inc.

Stockhausen, L. (1994). The clinical learning spiral: A model to develop reflective practitioners. *Nurse Education Today*, 14(5): 363–371.

Stockhausen, L. (2006). Métier artistry: Revealing reflection in action in everyday practice. *Nurse Education Today*, 26(1): 54–62.

Stockhausen, L. (2008). Learning to become a nurse: Students' reflections on their clinical experiences. *Australian Journal of Advanced Nursing*, 22(3): 8–14.

Stoerm, A. (2010). Reflective journaling 2.0: Using blogs to enhance experiential learning. *Journal of Nursing Education*, 49(10): 596.

Stuart, C.C. (2004). The use of a portfolio of clinical evidence to influence student learning in midwifery education. *Birth Issues*, 13(4): 121–127.

Taylor, B.J. (2010). *Reflective practice for healthcare professionals: A practical guide* (3rd ed.). Maidenhead, England: Open University Press.

Williams, M. & Watson, A. (2004). Post-lesson debriefing: delayed or immediate? An investigation of student teacher talk. *Journal of Education for Teaching*, 30(2): 85–96.

Zarezadeh, Y., Pearson, P. & Dickinson, C. (2009). A model for using reflection to enhance interprofessional education. *International Journal of Education*, 1(1): 1–18.

Zigmont, J., Kappus, L. & Sudikoff, S. (2011). The 3D model of debriefing: Defusing, discovering, and deepening. *Seminars in Perinatology*, 35(2): 52–58.

Developing Teaching and Learning

CHAPTER 8

Challenging Student Situations

KEY CONCEPTS

- Commonly encountered student situations
  - The unprofessional student
  - The reticent student
  - The unsafe student
  - Cultural and linguistic diversity
  - The exceptional student
  - The borderline or failing student
  - The overconfident student
- Dealing with challenging clinical issues
  - Death and dying
  - Smells and sights

INTRODUCTION

Teaching can be an interesting and rewarding venture because it enables encounters with a range of different students with different attributes. In most cases, learning and teaching episodes progress without any dilemmas arising. However, from time to time, situations appear that can be particularly challenging for the individual facilitating learning in practice.

A multitude of unique challenges surround learning for health professional students, particularly in clinical settings. Furthermore, some challenges can be multifactorial in nature, requiring careful and thoughtful handling. This chapter introduces some commonly encountered student situations in learning environments. It provides the means for identifying the issues and offers some support for the teacher attempting to handle them.

COMMONLY ENCOUNTERED STUDENT SITUATIONS

The Unprofessional Student

Unprofessional behaviour in some health professions is viewed as one aspect of not being fit for practice (McGurgan et al., 2010; Ellis et al., 2011). Students who display unprofessional behaviour may fail a clinical placement as a result of such an act. Unprofessionalism can appear in a range of student behaviours, some examples of which are listed in Table 8.1.

These types of behaviours can be particularly challenging for teachers and could be left unresolved for longer than they should be. Many course centres or universities now have established procedures for dealing with such student situations. Tact is necessary in dealing with many issues regarding unprofessional behaviour. This requires the teacher to quietly take the student into a private area where the behaviour of concern can be described.

TABLE 8.1 Characteristic Examples of the Unprofessional Student

- Arriving late to the practice or other setting
- Unethical behaviour regarding clients, their carers and family or other health professionals
- Dishonesty
- Lack of respect towards others in the professional setting
- Unacceptable or inappropriate personal presentation
- Non-adherence to professional guidelines or standards for practice
- Practices outside of accepted scope of practice
- Unprofessional verbal interchanges with clients or others
- Ignoring the boundaries of professional conduct

The student may be completely unaware that a problem exists, so in the first instance, the nature of the behaviour needs to be explained, along with the negative impact it might be having on the current clinical rotation as well as the potential impact on their future career. Referring to professional standards or guidelines for practice can provide a valuable resource for reinforcing expected behaviours. The student also needs the opportunity to respond to the criticism.

Next, it is important to set expected levels of performance for the student to achieve in order to rectify the problem, and a timeframe in which this is to happen. Following your verbal discussion together, these directions are best confirmed for the student in writing. If the problem is of a serious nature, it is important to involve academic staff from the university early in the process. Explicit documentation of the event as soon as possible after it occurs is needed in case such behaviours continue and the student fails the placement. This material will support a case for failure and provide a basis on which later remedial education can be provided.

ACTIVITY 8.1

Michael is a final-year health professional student who arrives to a scheduled team meeting 30 minutes late. It is his second day of placement. On entry to the meeting room he disrupts the discussion in progress by noisily finding a seat and then shuffling through a pile of papers. Michael appears shabbily dressed and his hair does not appear to have been combed. After the meeting is finished you need to address the situation with him. How will you approach it?

•••

The Reticent Student

Students may appear reticent to participate actively in the clinical setting for a number of reasons. They might fear making errors, failing the clinical rotation, hurting people, or being seen as a burden to staff; they might doubt their own capabilities or knowledge, or simply be shy or unmotivated. For others, reticence may be due to questioning whether their chosen profession is actually the right one for them, or be the result of personal circumstances impacting on their attention to the learning experience. While shyness may be overcome with time and experience, reticence due to other factors may lead to poor clinical performance (Murden et al., 2004). The reticent student may present in a range of different ways. Some examples are listed in Table 8.2.

Often reticent students are viewed as not interested and can attract disparaging remarks from other colleagues, but they might have a large number of concerns playing out in their minds. They may lack the necessary knowledge base to enact the experience, which may mean they are unsafe to be in the setting. The teacher

TABLE 8.2 Characteristic Examples of the Reticent Student

- Appearing disinterested in events happening in the practice setting
- Not eager to volunteer to undertake particular clinical tasks as opportunities arise
- Wanting to continually observe others perform clinical skills rather than doing them themselves
- Isolating themselves from their peers or student group
- Not engaging with clients without encouragement
- Not actively participating in group-learning sessions

needs to identify quickly the root cause of the student's hesitation, to allow the situation to be resolved and the student to progress satisfactorily through the experience. This requires the teacher to engage the student in a private discussion away from the physical learning environment, if possible, in a context of trust that encourages the student to reveal the cause of the problem. Once the cause is known, both teacher and student can work together to determine how best to address the situation. This may require setting some performance challenges to overcome an obstacle. For example, if the fear of harming a person is causing the problem, working through the fearful situation, with the teacher providing direct encouragement and support, may be all that is needed to overcome it. Where the situation is not easily and quickly rectified, university staff should be engaged to assist with planning an appropriate mode of action.

Often it may require a series of events to indicate a student's reticence to practise. Each of these events should be extensively documented as it occurs. In some instances documentation will record only one isolated event. However, in other cases, a series of documentation will provide a solid foundation on which to make a judgement about the student's ability to achieve a satisfactory outcome. It also provides evidence on which academic staff may implement remedial action should that be required.

ACTIVITY 8.2

Sophie is a second-year student who has been in your unit for the past week. While Sophie can implement appropriate care when prompted, she appears to lack self-direction. Her knowledge base appears sound, although she is not keen to share this openly. In her interactions with clients, she appears to have difficulty engaging in conversation. As Sophie's clinical teacher, how might you begin to improve this situation?

The Unsafe Student

Clinical teachers contribute to both student performance and the safety of clients in students' care (Glavin, 2006). Recognising an unsafe student is, therefore, an important responsibility. The unsafe student is one who practises in a haphazard or potentially dangerous way or who practises outside their scope, which possibly risks client safety. Often this student does not possess the requisite theory underpinning clinical practice but continues to engage in hands-on clinical work. In other cases, the student may present to the clinical setting impaired by drugs and/or alcohol, or display signs of mental impairment.

In these situations the clinical teacher needs to take prompt action with the unsafe student in order to ensure client safety. Initially, this requires removing the student from the immediate clinical situation. In private, the student needs to be informed of the unsafe nature of their work. During this discussion it is useful to explore with the student their understanding of underlying theory, to evaluate whether the unsafe practice relates either to a knowledge deficit, an incongruous attitude or another factor. In the vast majority of cases the teacher will need to include university staff in rectifying the problem. This may require preparing additional remedial theory preparation and/or additional practice in a simulated environment where client safety is not threatened until the student is able to demonstrate a safe level of knowledge and practice.

Precise and extensive documentation is required that details the context in which the safety issue was identified. Where applicable, this documentation should seek to link the unsafe actions to the relevant professional standards or competencies.

ACTIVITY 8.3

Joyce is a second-year student with whom you have been working for the past two days. Initially, you were concerned that Joyce's knowledge base did not appear to be at the level required and have since been observing her practice. This morning you are called by clinical staff members who tell you that Joyce has undertaken a clinical procedure without supervision. Staff members are also concerned as they believe Joyce may not yet have had instruction in the procedure. You confirm this to be the case. What will you do?

....

Cultural and Linguistic Diversity

The number of students from culturally and linguistically diverse (CALD) backgrounds is increasing in health professional courses (Salamonson et al., 2012). Some CALD students have been born in the country where they are studying, while others were not. Some have well-developed communication skills, while others do not. Within this group, a range of significant differences might arise and CALD students may experience individual difficulties in the clinical setting. Language and communication is a problem for some of these learners, while others find local cultural practices to be new and confronting to their own backgrounds. Many may also be unfamiliar with western approaches to healthcare. Facilitating learning for CALD students is covered in more detail in Chapter 2. Practice problems that may arise for CALD learners include:

- Speaking, listening and being understood
- Understanding medical terminology
- Feeling uncomfortable about asking questions
- Encountering racism and prejudice
- Understanding the scope of practice
- Adjusting to different nursing practices and local cultures.

It is important for the teacher to establish relationships with students on commencement of their placement, to facilitate its success and provide ongoing support and encouragement, especially where communication skills are developing. Helpful strategies may include the following:

- Promote an environment where students feel comfortable, and are permitted, to ask questions.

- Support students in their interactions with health professionals and clients to promote confidence in their communication skills.
- Support students during clinical practice where cultural boundaries and practices are different to what they are accustomed.
- Find another student or health professional mentor from a similar background who can assist with their socialisation and learning.
- Encourage reading in English (such as newspapers) and watching locally produced television to refine reading and listening skills (it is useful to ask the student to report back the next day on their activities).
- Promote reflective journaling written in English throughout the learning experience.
- Ask students to develop questions to pose at the end of each day.

Remedios and Webb (2005) suggest that, where communication skills may be problematic, clinical teachers evaluate them early in the placement by setting tasks focused on communication. In addition, they suggest using paraphrasing and questioning to promote correct interpretations.

ACTIVITY 8.4

Li is a first-year international student who is having her first clinical placement with you. All is progressing well until you encounter an elderly Caucasian client who refuses to have Li involved in his care because of her cultural background. Understandably, Li becomes distressed by the client's rejection of her. How will you handle this situation? It should also be noted that not all communication problems stem from cultural and linguistic diversities.

The Exceptional Student

Exceptionality is a very broad term used to identify difference from the normal or mainstream. In educational contexts, this may refer to gifted students or those with learning or other disabilities. Little, if anything, is written about the academically advanced or gifted student in the health professions. However, teaching a student of this nature has the potential to be as challenging as working with one who is struggling. This student can be intimidating for the teacher, demanding additional learning opportunities than other students. On the other hand, the student may appear bored or frustrated, or may fear failing the placement (Foster, 2007). It is particularly important for these students to be challenged in both the classroom and in practice learning environments. This may require the teacher to develop additional learning activities to keep the learner motivated. Providing support and reassurance where the student is fearful of failing the placement may also be necessary.

A range of learning disabilities exist and these should not be detrimental to the successful completion of a clinical placement or course. However, the individualisation of learning activities may require the teacher to be more creative than normal in selecting learning opportunities and providing additional support. Usually course centres or universities have disability support units that can provide invaluable guidance with successfully managing such students.

Recent studies in the health professions describe there are students with dyslexia or those who have 'a difficulty with language' (Sanderson-Mann & McCandless, 2006, p. 128). While such difficulties are specific to the individual case, Sanderson-Mann and McCandless (2006) identify that dyslexic nursing students may have difficulty with written or verbal communication, time management and documentation. These authors argue that such students require a supportive learning environment, individualised strategies, and an understanding faculty that readily accepts them despite their difficulties. Foster (2008) reaffirms the need to tailor individual learning experiences based on the learner's strengths and weaknesses, as they should be for any learner.

ACTIVITY 8.5

John is a final-year student who has been working with you for the past week. He is confident and has an excellent clinical skill and theoretical knowledge base. John is able to complete set tasks to a high standard and in a very timely manner. However, he complains to you he is not feeling stimulated, is bored and does not feel he is learning enough on the placement. How will you respond to this?

The Borderline or Failing Student

Dealing with the borderline or failing student is challenging and often time consuming for teachers, particularly in clinical areas. Research has indicated that clinical teachers find it very difficult to fail students. Many hesitate and will seek ways to pass the student (Adams & Adamson, 2004) rather than confront the reality that the student should not pass. Sometimes clinical teachers may perceive the failing student as a failure on their part, doubting their own abilities (Rutkowski, 2007). At other times, wanting to avoid confronting the student with the negative news of their results leads clinical teachers to pass a student who has not performed to a satisfactory level. All situations of failure are difficult and can challenge the teacher's own self-confidence (Jervis & Tilki, 2011).

Dealing with a failing student in clinical learning environments can be complex. In the health professions, it is important to discriminate between needing to care for the student's wellbeing and the professional responsibility that being a clinical teacher entails. It is important to remember that professional standards, used to assess performance, are in place to develop competent health professionals. Needlessly passing a student who has not reached the required level puts at risk professional standards as well as public safety. Furthermore, it does not allow for underlying problems to be addressed, leading to substandard practices being taken into subsequent clinical placements or graduate practice. However, there are also repercussions for students. Having to perform competently during practice placements is extremely stressful for some students. Failure may result in needing to repeat a year of the course and further personal and financial stress to achieve this (Emerson, 2007).

For the borderline or failing student to successfully complete a practice placement, it can require an extensive investment of time and energy on the part of the clinical teacher in coaching and supporting the student. However, this is not impossible if the situation is identified early and assistive measures are quickly put in place. The teacher needs to work closely with the student to foster growth rather than distancing themselves (McGregor, 2007). Including colleagues in decision making will provide the teacher with needed support and guidance during the process (Luhanga et al., 2008). The following strategies may assist with managing the borderline or failing student:

- Identify the student's particular deficits. These should be extensively documented as they become evident.
- Determine the measures needed to address the student's deficits successfully.
- Determine if there is sufficient time and resources available to address the deficits alongside the learning experience.
- Determine if the student is unsafe. If so, they are best removed from the placement to rectify their issues through remedial work within the university context.
- Seek guidance from academic staff throughout the process to confirm the most appropriate strategy.
- Redistribute the amount of time spent with other students on the placement to allow sufficient time to work with the borderline student.
- Set clearly defined clinical challenges that the student must reach in allocated time periods.
- Avoid standing over the student, which causes intimidation and fear that impairs their ability to practise.
- Provide feedback in such a way that it allows direction for personal and/or professional growth.
- Ensure that you remain objective in assessing the student.
- Document progress against the challenge criteria.

ACTIVITY 8.6

Amanda is a student with whom you have been working for the past two weeks. She appears to have a sound grasp of the theoretical principles underpinning her practice. However, Amanda is struggling with hands-on skills, making it difficult for her to achieve her required competencies for the placement. You are concerned that she may not be able to pass the placement as a result but want to support her. From your observations, she appears to have difficulty with dexterity. How might you approach this situation?

The Overconfident Student

Overconfident students may also be encountered in clinical learning environments. While confidence is important to clinical practice, overconfidence can be problematic and potentially risky.

The overconfident student usually appears to possess a very sound knowledge base that contributes to the levels of confidence played out in the setting. In some instances the student may be acting in an overconfident manner to impress the teacher who is also responsible for the placement assessment. However, research suggests that overconfidence can interfere with effective decision making and can lead to potential errors (Berner & Graber, 2008; Smith & Agate, 2004). Therefore, the ramifications of allowing a student to practise in an overconfident manner could be detrimental.

The overconfident student may be difficult to constrain; however, the teacher has a responsibility for client safety. Where a student is overconfident, the teacher needs to meet privately with the student to present the issues and potential ramifications. It is also important to praise the student's very sound theoretical knowledge base but repeat educational and professional boundaries. Following the meeting, working alongside the student for some time can be useful in assisting them to progress through the clinical decision-making process in a careful, systematic and accurate way. This can aid the student in identifying where their practice had previously been moving too fast and work towards rectifying their overconfidence.

Paula is a second-year student with whom you are working to provide care to an allocated client. She confidently approaches the tasks at hand, completing them quickly and efficiently; then she progresses to the needs of another client. However, in delivering care to the first client she fails to recognise he has developed a raised respiratory rate. What actions will you take?

DEALING WITH CHALLENGING CLINICAL ISSUES

Death and Dying

Death and dying are almost always difficult for health professional students to deal with but, for most, these events are a reality of the nature of the work in which they engage. For many students a clinical placement might be the first time they encounter death and dying. Others may have previously experienced losing a grandparent or other loved one. Students may have received some theory around death and dying in the classroom, but less experience in the realities of practice. Regardless, the first encounter with death and dying in practice is likely to evoke an array of emotional responses.

The teacher plays a key role in ensuring support for students who encounter death and dying. Within some healthcare settings, students may not be engaged in the direct care of clients who are dying; however, they may be equally distressed to learn that a client whom they had previously cared for has died.

Regardless of the level of involvement, it is important to assess each learner for support with grieving. For those students who are able to engage in direct care, many skills may be acquired for their future practice if they are allowed to provide care in a supported environment. Allowing for this type of opportunity requires teachers to be readily available and aware of the students' needs. Strategies for supporting a student caring for clients who are dying may include the following:

- Encourage the student to write about their own feelings surrounding death and dying and continue to document their reflections.
- Work with the student to explore their own meanings around death.
- Provide explicit detail for the student prior to engaging with the client, with regard to diagnosis, prognosis and physical, psycho-social and spiritual needs.
- Prepare the student for what to expect when they enter the room.
- Involve the student in team meetings with other health professionals involved in the client's care.
- Encourage and provide direct support for the student participating in care for the dying or deceased person.
- Debrief the student and assess their emotional status regularly.
- Allow the student to participate in the care of the client who has died if they wish to.
- Work with students to understand the responses of the client's family.
- Identify additional support mechanisms for the student such as a chaplain or counselling service.

ACTIVITY 8.8

Most health professionals can readily recall their first encounter with death and dying. They can recollect the client, the situation, how they felt and the support they received in coping. Recall your own first encounter. Consider the support you received. Did it address your needs?

Determine how would you now support a learner through a similar encounter.

Smells and Sights

Students in the health professions encounter a vast array of conditions afflicting the human body. Some of these can be particularly confronting. Strange smells and sights are commonly encountered in practice settings such as disfigurement (as a result of burns, amputation, wounds or congenital malformation), and offensive odours (such as those related to melaena or a grossly infected wound).

Initial encounters with such confronting situations can be particularly distressing for students as they attempt to manage their own feelings and physical responses to such situations. However, for health professionals who have encountered them many times before, their response may be so attuned they no longer react. The way in which initial encounters are handled is likely to have a lasting impact on the learner. Facial responses evoked by the student may have a potential effect on the client's self-concept. Hence, such situations should be handled carefully and tactfully.

The teacher plays an important role in assisting students to work effectively with their personal feelings in order to deliver appropriate client care. Preparing the student prior to entering the client's room is a first step in providing support. Explain in detail the nature of the disfigurement or odour. At this point, graphic details will allow the student to create a picture in their mind and begin to deal with their feelings. Discuss how facial and other responses need to be controlled in order to reduce the impact on the client. O'Connor (2006) suggests having students identify something to focus on, such as the client's eyes, and entering dialogue with the client quickly to remove the focus on the disfigurement or odour. It is important throughout the care episode for the teacher to stay with the student, providing ongoing support.

Visions of a disfigurement may linger in a student's mind for some time. On leaving the client's room, it is important to provide opportunities for the student to debrief on their encounter. Provide opportunities to discuss the student's feelings and reactions. Should the student require support beyond the clinical placement, refer the situation to university academic staff to ensure the student receives the appropriate follow-up care.

ACTIVITY 8.9

Reflect on a situation where, as a student, you had an initial encounter with disfigurement or a particularly offensive smell. What were your initial reactions?

How did you handle the situation?

What support did you receive?

Document how you would, as the teacher, support a student having that experience for the first time.

⟦⊙⟧ SNAPSHOT

Teaching in the health professions can present many challenges when different types of student situations arise. By being at the forefront of supporting students in their learning, the teacher is central to identifying issues as they appear, developing strategies for dealing with them and supporting students through difficult experiences. This chapter presents some of the common situations encountered by teachers, particularly in the practice setting. Despite this, it is impossible to cover all of the possibilities in such an unpredictable role. However, the overarching principles for managing such situations involve remaining objective, constructive and learner centred.

REFERENCES AND FURTHER READING

Adams, E.J. & Adamson, B.J. (2004). Evaluation of the borderline student: An allied health perspective. *Focus on Health Professional Education: A Multidisciplinary Journal*, 6(2): 11–21.

Berner, E.S. & Graber, M.L. (2008). Overconfidence as a cause of diagnostic error in medicine. *American Journal of Medicine*, 121(5 Suppl.): S2–S23.

Ellis, J., Lee-Woolf, E. & David, T. (2011). Supporting nursing students during fitness to practice hearings. *Nursing Standard*, 25(32): 38–43.

Emerson, R.J. (2007). *Nursing education in the clinical setting*. St Louis: Mosby Elsevier.

Foster, I. (2008). Enhancing the learning experience of student radiographers with dyslexia. *Radiography*, 14(1): 32–38.

Foster, J. (2007). Cultivating giftedness: How parents and teachers can support exceptional learners. *Orbit*, 7(1): 36–38.

Glavin, R. (2006). What every clinical teacher should know about patient safety. *The Clinical Teacher*, 3(2): 103–106.

Jervis, A. & Tilki, M. (2011). Why are nurse mentors failing to fail student nurses who do not meet clinical performance standards? *British Journal of Nursing*, 20(9): 582–587.

Kraemer Tebes, J., Matlin, S.L., Migdole, S.J., Farkas, M.S., Money, R.W., Shulman, L. & Hoge, M.A. (2011). Providing competency training to clinical supervisors through an instructional supervision approach. *Research on Social Work Practice*, 21(2): 190–199.

Luhanga, F., Yonge, O. & Myrick, F. (2008). Precepting an unsafe student: The role of faculty. *Nurse Education Today*, 28(2): 227–231.

McGregor, A. (2007). Academic success, clinical failure: Struggling practices of a failing student. *Journal of Nursing Education*, 46(11): 504–510.

McGurgan, P.M., Olson-White, D., Holgate, M. & Carmody, D. (2010). Fitness-to-practise policies in Australian medical schools: Are they fit for purpose? *Medical Journal of Australia*, 193(11): 665–667.

Murden, R.A., Way, D.P., Hudson, A. & Westman, J.A. (2004). Professionalism deficiencies in a first-quarter doctor–patient relationship course predict poor clinical performance in medical school. *Academic Medicine*, 79(10 Suppl.): S46–S48.

O'Connor, A.B. (2006). *Clinical instruction and evaluation: A teaching resource* (2nd ed.). Boston: Jones and Bartlett.

Remedios, L. & Webb, G. (2005). Clinical educators as cultural guides. In R. Rose & D. Best (Eds), *Transforming practice through clinical education, professional supervision and mentoring* (pp. 207–218). Edinburgh: Elsevier.

Rutkowski, K. (2007). Failure to fail: Assessing nursing students' competence during practice placement. *Nursing Standard*, 22(13): 35–40.

Salamonson, Y., Ramjan, L., Lombardo, L., Lanser, L., Fernandez, R. & Griffiths, R. (2012). Diversity and demographic heterogeneity of Australian nursing students: A closer look. *International Nursing Review*, 59(1): 59–65.

Sanderson-Mann, J. & McCandless, F. (2006). Understanding dyslexia and nurse education in the clinical setting. *Nurse Education in Practice*, 6(1): 127–133.

Smith, J.D. & Agate, J. (2004). Solutions for overconfidence: Evaluation of an instructional module for counselor trainees. *Counselor Education & Supervision*, 44(1): 31–43.

CHAPTER 9

Developing as a Teacher

KEY CONCEPTS

- Roles and responsibilities
- Managing time and workload
- Identifying and managing 'hidden curricula'
- Managing complex interpersonal relationships
- Reflective practice and self-care
- Professional development
- Using a professional teaching portfolio
- Mentoring

INTRODUCTION

Previous chapters have explored many practical aspects of effective teaching and learning. This chapter takes a different direction and focuses attention on the teacher. The first part looks at some of the challenges faced by teachers in their daily work such as time management and interpersonal relationships. Teachers may act in their roles intermittently or may be seeking to make their role a permanent one. The second part of the chapter focuses on developing as a teacher and explores strategies for enhancing professional role development. Such aspects include the role of reflective practice to develop expertise, developing a professional teaching portfolio, seeking out resources and considering a mentor.

ROLES AND RESPONSIBILITIES

Chapter 1 examines the fundamental roles and responsibilities of being a teacher in the health professions. These include having the capabilities and characteristics of a role model, teacher, assessor, supervisor, coach, client advocate, motivator and resource director. Discussions in previous chapters show how these responsibilities are multifaceted: the teacher has responsibilities towards students and their learning, the university, clients and their families, other health professionals, healthcare organisations and the profession itself more broadly. Thus the areas that clinical teachers have responsibility for are highly complex and may include:
- Student teaching and learning outcomes
- Student and client safety
- Quality of care
- Advocacy for students and clients
- Effective relationships among members of the healthcare team
- Effective communication between all stakeholders
- Professional, ethical and legal values and standards.

ACTIVITY 9.1

Consider your own teaching work. List the responsibilities you recognise within the role. What strategies do you employ to meet those responsibilities?

Are there aspects of these responsibilities that you could develop further?

MANAGING TIME AND WORKLOAD

Teaching can be like performing a juggling act, in which time plays a significant role. In clinical settings, some teachers will be responsible for a number of students while others may have responsibility for just one or two but may also carry a clinical caseload. Hence, meeting all of the different responsibilities can be challenging. In addition, different types of teaching are likely to be performed. For example, just-in-time teaching occurs in an ad hoc fashion and is usually based on providing direct client care in the clinical setting (Hoffman & Donaldson, 2004). Making the most of these brief encounters requires effective questioning to optimise the experience. The One Minute Preceptor model reported by Neher et al. (1992) is widely advocated to facilitate these clinical encounters. The model has five steps:

1. *Get a commitment*: Explore with the learner their interpretation of the clinical situation.
2. *Probe for supporting evidence*: Allow time to understand what the learner does and does not know about the situation.
3. *Teach general rules*: Discuss aspects that can be taken from the situation and applied in similar situations.
4. *Reinforce what was done correctly*: Allow for positive feedback and promote self-esteem.
5. *Correct mistakes*: Offer constructive feedback and improvement suggestions. (Kertis, 2007; Molodysky, 2007)

In addition to ad hoc teaching encounters, clinical teachers may include formalised teaching and learning sessions outside of the clinical area such as debriefing or tutorial sessions. The latter require quarantined periods during the clinical day. Ideally they are organised for quieter periods so that students will not miss out on important clinical learning opportunities.

Time pressures in teaching can emanate from a range of influences. Clinical teachers sometimes find themselves trying to balance spending equitable time with each student, and attempting to provide additional support for those students requiring it to meet their clinical learning objectives. This may be influenced by the perception of needing to be a supervisor of student activity rather than a facilitator of student learning (McKenna, 2004). Hence, having a clear understanding of your own role in supporting students in their learning is important, as well as incorporating other factors such as the need to provide client care. While it has been argued that working with a student reduces clinical productivity, Berger et al. (2004) conclude in their medical study that achieving a balance between sound client care and clinical teaching effectiveness is possible.

One way of organising the teaching workload in the clinical setting is to develop a daily plan that incorporates a number of different variables. The variables may include the detailed use of diaries and calendars, or more formalised tools such as Gantt charts. While careful workload planning is important, the dynamic nature of the learning environment means that plans do need to change at certain times. However, factors that should be considered in organising clinical teaching workload on a daily basis include:

- Student learning objectives
- Key priorities for client care
- Student capacity to assist with client care
- Geographical location/s of students
- Individual student learning requirements and progress towards these.

For clinical teachers assuming responsibility for a number of students spread out across a venue, it can be particularly difficult to manage time effectively. It is also impossible to be with each student all of the time. The following strategies may be useful in organising time and monitoring student learning in such situations:

- Include other clinicians in providing student support as much as possible. Ensure they understand the level of student preparation and their learning needs and that they are willing to support the student. Seek regular feedback from clinicians working with students.
- Review the clients each student will be working with each day. Reinforce with students the types of clinical activities you wish to work on with them directly, so they may call you when these arise.
- Try to allocate some direct time for each student each day, knowing there will be some students who are likely to require more input from you than others. This will require some flexibility to allow for managing unexpected events.
- Have students maintain a log of their activities during the day. You can review these to get a picture of their activities and learning while you were not present. They can also provide prompts for questions to explore each student's learning when opportunities do become available.
- Maintain a log of the activities you undertake with each student over the duration of the placement. This will help ensure that each student meets their clinical learning requirements and will allow for the monitoring of individual development.

ACTIVITY 9.2

Reflect on your own time management. What are some of the challenges you face in managing your clinical teaching and other workloads?

What strategies do you use to prioritise demands?

IDENTIFYING AND MANAGING THE HIDDEN CURRICULA

The concept of the existence of 'hidden curricula' has been identified in many disciplines. It has been argued that some professional values are taught and learnt through unintended processes, 'informal' (Thiedke, 2004) or 'de facto' curricula (Sambell & McDowell, 1998). What students witness in clinical practice can have a powerful impact on the development of their professional behaviours (Glicken & Merenstein, 2007). In contrast to intended curriculum outcomes, hidden curricula may be enforced through clinicians and others having expectations of learners outside of those formally intended, through implicit messages or agendas that students reinforce.

McKenna (2004) interviewed nursing clinical teachers about their roles and identified that hidden or 'personal curricula' underpinned their clinical teaching. These curricula were created by teachers themselves around what they considered students needed to be able to do and know within clinical environments, such as individual performance expectations at each year level of the course. Overall, discourses informing the 'personal curricula' were imbedded in clinical practice, with their emphasis on 'doing' and teaching centred on clinical practice and practical skills development. These curricula had the potential to undermine the intended academic curriculum expectations and cause conflict for students seeking to meet two different sets of clinical practice expectations.

Hidden curricula are complex entities. With different influences on students during their clinical learning, it is impossible to eliminate all agendas outside the formal curriculum. While many of these can have a negative influence, some may actually be positive for student development. For the clinical teacher it is important to recognise the multitude of influences impacting on the students' development during their placements, and to work with them to sort through different experiences and draw out positive influences. From here, students can be guided into discriminating what they see and experience in order to develop effective professional behaviours.

ACTIVITY 9.3

Reflect on the assumptions or expectations you bring to your own clinical teaching role. What are they?

What has influenced their development?

Are the assumptions and expectations imbedded in students' academic curricula?

Do these influence your expectations of students' performances in clinical placements?

Are they beneficial to students' learning and practice outcomes?

MANAGING COMPLEX INTERPERSONAL RELATIONSHIPS

Teachers, especially those in clinical settings, draw on a complex array of skills to establish and maintain interpersonal relationships with students. These can include nurturing, advocating, supporting, guiding and supervising relationships. However, student relationships represent only one aspect. Teaching effectiveness in practice environments requires quality interactions with a number of other groups, including:

- Different health professional staff across the clinical agency
- Hospital administrators
- Clients and their families
- University staff (academic and administrative).

Clinical teachers are commonly engaged by universities to undertake their teaching roles at other, clinically-based locations. This has the potential to create tensions if demands from the health provider come into conflict with the university's requirements. Sometimes it is easy for the teacher to forget they are employed by a university rather than a healthcare agency due to where they are performing their teaching role. In other cases clinical teachers are employed by health providers and either add student teaching to their existing clinical workload, or they are seconded temporarily from clinical responsibilities to assume clinical teaching work. For those clinical teachers who carry clinical workloads as well as teaching ones, there is also the potential for tension between meeting their clients' care needs and meeting students' learning requirements. Hence, care needs to be taken to ensure these are balanced.

It is important to remember that sound relationships within the teaching and learning environment are paramount to facilitating learning. In the clinical setting these relationships can ease students' access to necessary clinical experiences. Hence, diplomacy becomes an important function. Within each group exists different personalities, genders and cultural backgrounds. These all need to be managed carefully to ensure students' learning experiences are positive and they are able to meet their learning requirements.

ACTIVITY 9.4

Consider your own teaching practice. List the groups of people with whom you commonly interact in one day. Which ones have the potential to influence student learning?

What strategies do you employ to ensure your interpersonal relationships are positive?

REFLECTIVE PRACTICE AND SELF-CARE

Reflective practice is discussed comprehensively in Chapter 7. It is reinforced here because it has become a vital part of professional practice. Health professional curricula expect students and graduates to be capable of reflective practice. For clinical teachers, reflective practice offers great opportunities to develop the many components of their role and for professional growth. To extend ideas of reflection further, Johns (2004, p. 3) describes it as:

... being mindful of self, either within or after experience, as if a window through which the practitioner can view and focus self within the context of a particular experience, in order to confront, understand and move toward resolving contradiction between one's vision and actual practice. Through the conflict of contradiction, the commitment to realise one's vision, and understanding why things are as they are, the practitioner can gain new insights into self and be empowered to respond more congruently in future situations within a reflexive spiral towards developing practical wisdom and realising one's vision as a lived reality.

Fundamentally, reflective practice revolves around examining one's own experiences, integrating this knowledge in order to enhance both understanding and the development of practice. Schon (1983) describes two different types of reflection: reflection-in-action and reflection-on-action. As the names infer, reflection-in-action relates to reflection undertaken in the process of care delivery, while reflection-on-action occurs retrospectively and this allows for deeper understanding and growth to occur. It provides opportunities to explore knowledge and feelings surrounding the particular activity (Lau et al., 2002).

There are strategies by which clinical teachers can reflect effectively on their practice. Similar to students, individual reflective journals, diaries and logs provide opportunities for written self-reflection, critical-incident analysis and professional growth (Johns, 2010). Peer reflection with other clinical teachers can also facilitate reflective practice. Sharing clinical teaching experiences with others can enhance learning and allow for different perspectives and interpretations to be considered, facilitating professional growth for all group members. Taylor (2010) advocates having a 'critical friend' who can listen while you share your practice reflections and help interpret and make sense of them. The sharing of experiences in secure online discussion forums can also assist clinical teachers. These forums help develop a sense of 'not being alone'; they can reaffirm creative approaches to student learning and provide constructive advice on challenging encounters.

ACTIVITY 9.5

Reflect on one of your significant teaching episodes, such as providing a student with feedback. Write about the experience and what you have learnt as a result. Would you act differently if the situation arose again? You can also use the reflective practice framework in Learning Resource 5 to help interrogate your learning.

The role of teacher or practice partner can be complex and challenging. Health professionals regularly incorporate supporting learners with their clinical loads, and those in academia have other requirements to fulfil such as research and community engagement. Hence, teaching has the potential to be demanding, stressful, and lead to burnout. Therefore it is important to take the time to incorporate self-care strategies into your daily life. Engaging in reflective practice is one way to achieve this, through such activities as journaling, debriefing with others, or practising mindfulness. O'Connor (2011) suggests that sharing responsibilities with others, along with making the time to engage in healthy lifestyle activities outside of the work environment, are effective strategies. Lifestyle activities may include hobbies, sports participation, meditation, taking regular holidays, or spending time with family and friends.

ACTIVITY 9.6

Reflect on the self-care strategies you currently use. Are they effective?

What other strategies could you consider to ensure you manage your own wellbeing?

PROFESSIONAL DEVELOPMENT

Ongoing professional development for all teachers is important to ensure the highest quality of teaching and learning. It facilitates access to up-to-date knowledge and practice around teaching and learning. It also has the potential to impact on attitudes towards teaching and learning (Steinert, 2005). However, with their isolation from others, clinical teachers may feel there are limited opportunities for professional development to assist with their role development. A range of opportunities does exist, but those chosen will depend on your long-term goals in education (Hays, 2007). Hence it is important to consider what educational roles you are planning for the future.

Steinert (2005) suggests a number of strategies by which clinical teachers can undertake relevant professional development in order to enhance their role, including attending workshops, seminars and conferences. Postgraduate studies provide a formal mechanism for developing skills and knowledge around education. A number of generic graduate diploma and masters programs are currently available in health professional and clinical education institutions throughout Australia and New Zealand. These directly provide theory and practice to develop teaching expertise for health professionals. Many other courses dealing with education are also available within specific disciplines, such as in medicine and nursing. At a higher-degree level, doctoral programs provide research training through which one can undertake projects on a multitude of topics, including aspects surrounding clinical education.

Engaging with professional journals is another way of participating in relevant professional development. There is a range of journals that focuses specifically on education in one or more of the health professions. Such journals contain up-to-date educational research that can be used to develop and enhance clinical teaching. In addition, many generic journals regularly include education-related articles. Table 9.1 presents some of the relevant journals that may be initial useful resources.

TABLE 9.1 Journals Specifically Focusing on Health Professional Education

Health Professionals

Advances in Health Sciences Education

Education for Health: Change in Learning and Practice

Focus on Health Professional Education: A Multidisciplinary Journal

International Journal of Clinical Skills

Journal for Continuing Education in the Health Professions

Journal of Dental Education

Simulation in Healthcare

The Clinical Teacher

Work Based Learning in Primary Care

Medicine

Academic Medicine

BMC Medical Education

Internet Journal of Medical Simulation

Medical Education

Medical Teacher

Teaching and Learning in Medicine: An International Journal

Nursing

Clinical Simulation in Nursing

Journal for Nurses in Staff Development

Journal of Continuing Education in Nursing

Nurse Education in Practice

Nurse Education Today

Nurse Educator

Nursing Education Perspectives

Online Journal of Nursing Education Scholarship

Teaching and Learning in Nursing

While the options are fairly limited, there are also professional organisations that focus specifically on health professional education. Joining one of these organisations offers opportunities to engage with other health professionals who have a particular affinity for education. Table 9.2 provides examples of some of the current options.

Furthermore, there are many evidence-based learning and teaching resources available to teachers on the Internet. Many of these resources offer quick references to particular areas of interest and can add to your repertoire of understanding student learning and teaching approaches and strategies.

TABLE 9.2 Professional Organisations with a Specific Education Focus

Association for the Study of Medical Education (ASME)	www.asme.org.uk/
Association for Medical Education in Europe (AMEE)	www.amee.org/index.asp?tm=22
Australia and New Zealand Association for Health Professional Educators (ANZAHPE)	http://anzahpe.org/
Australian Nurse Teachers Society	www.ants.org.au
Australian Rural Health Education Network	www.arhen.org.au/
Australian Society for Simulation in Healthcare	www.simulationaustralia.org.au/divisions/about-assh
Federation of Rural Australian Medical Educators (FRAME)	http://som.flinders.edu.au/FUSA/GP-Evidence/rural/frame/
International Nursing Association for Clinical Simulation and Learning	www.inacsl.org/INACSL_2010/
International Society of Educators in Physiotherapy	www.wcpt.org/node/24947
Society for Simulation in Healthcare	http://ssih.org/

ACTIVITY 9.7

Consider your needs for professional development. Construct a set of short- and long-term objectives relating to your teaching practice. What types of professional development options will you require to achieve these objectives?

••

USING A PROFESSIONAL TEACHING PORTFOLIO

With the move by many health professions towards credentialing and mandated continuing professional development, the use of professional portfolios has grown over recent years. Chapter 4 describes how a learning portfolio can be useful for students to demonstrate their learning achievements. In a similar way, portfolios provide a tool by which professional activities of teachers can be tracked and evidence retained. Andre and Heartfield (2011) define a professional portfolio as 'a structured collection of different types of information and evidence that show the individual's continuing professional development activities and experiences, competencies, and professional achievements and goals' (p. 4). In promoting lifelong learning, a professional portfolio progressively collects information across an individual's career.

For a health professional engaged in teaching activities, a teaching portfolio may constitute a component of a larger clinically-related portfolio. Xu (2004) suggests that a 'teaching portfolio is an organised collection of evidence about a teacher's best work that is selective, reflective and collaborative' (p. 199). Teaching portfolios provide opportunities to undertake personal reflections and to record teaching experiences as well as personal goals and priorities for the future.

Teaching portfolios can be developed in many ways, although commonly these are divided into particular sections that present different aspects. Ouellett (2007) suggests starting a teaching portfolio with a statement around one's personal teaching philosophy and perceptions around teaching. For a clinical teacher's portfolio, this is a good place to begin. This is aptly followed by a learning plan consisting of both short- and long-term goals or objectives related to teaching practice (Thistlethwaite, 2006).

A collection of teaching evidence is important, to support claims of your activities and engagement as well as provide a foundation on which to build further personal and professional development. The collected evidence specific to clinical teaching is diverse and might include the:

- Characteristics of students taught, including the dates or hours, numbers of students, year levels and areas of focus
- Curriculum details, including the synopsis and objectives of the academic unit in which the learning experience was placed, as well as any specific clinical learning objectives
- Methods of assessment used, both formal and informal
- Student feedback such as 'thank you' notes, letters or formal teacher evaluations
- Personal reflections on specific teaching and learning encounters, including both positive and less-positive teaching experiences
- Details of formal teaching presentations delivered
- Peer reviews of teaching encounters
- Self-appraisals and reflections of teaching.

ACTIVITY 9.8

Reflect on your own teaching experience. What aspects could you incorporate into a teaching portfolio?

How might you organise the supporting data?

What is the philosophy of teaching and learning that underpins your teaching?

What are the long- and short-term goals for your teaching work?

MENTORING

Mentoring can be a valuable process to support professional development for teachers in the health professions. However, much confusion exists around this role. Commonly the term 'mentoring' is incorrectly employed to refer to a model for the provision of clinical teaching, and is sometimes confused with 'coaching'. Mentoring has been described as relating 'primarily to the identification and nurturing of potential for the whole person' (Megginson & Clutterbuck, 2005, p. 4). Unlike other relationships, mentoring can be long term.

Over time mentoring has been viewed as involving a relationship between an older, experienced mentor in the field in which the mentee was developing. Given the complex, and often solitary, nature of clinical teaching, mentoring offers opportunities to engage in relationships that foster professional role development, career advice and feedback. However, the success of the relationship hinges on communication styles, commitment levels and the nature of the relationship itself.

Finding a mentor requires careful consideration. The mentor must be able to assist you with meeting your professional goals, so these should underpin your search. White and Tryon (2007, p. 1258) provide some key questions to consider when making this decision, including:

- Do you feel admiration for the person as a professional?
- Are they currently engaged or have been in the type of role you would like to pursue?
- Do they attract respect from their colleagues?
- Do they have a positive disposition, an optimistic approach and enthusiasm towards their work?
- Are you comfortable enough with them to allow for personal discussions?
- Can you trust your discussions will be held in confidence?
- Will you be able to accept challenges and candidness from them?
- Are you ready to enter into a mentoring relationship?

ACTIVITY 9.9

Reflect on your own career development. What are your goals with regard to teaching?

How might a mentoring relationship assist your work as a teacher?

What would you be looking for in a mentor?

From the criteria above, try to identify a person who would make an effective mentor for you.

⟨◎⟩ SNAPSHOT

This chapter revisits some of the complexity inherent in teaching in the health professions. Issues such as time management, managing the hidden curricula and interpersonal relationships are explored specifically in the context of clinical teaching work. As highlighted, these are not straightforward issues but the reader has been encouraged to explore strategies to assist with managing them.

The chapter also discusses the importance of professional development in what can often be a solitary role. Reflective practice and maintaining a professional teaching portfolio are reinforced because they allow for the development of teaching expertise. Finding resources for developing teaching practice will also be of benefit. The importance of finding a suitable mentor who can provide a sounding board and offer advice can be a highly valuable component in developing as a teacher.

REFERENCES AND FURTHER READING

Andre, K. & Heartfield, M. (2011). *Nursing and midwifery portfolios: Evidence of continuing competence* (2nd ed.). Sydney: Churchill Livingstone Elsevier.

Aultman, J.M. (2005). Uncovering the hidden medical curriculum through a pedagogy of discomfort. *Advances in Health Sciences Education*, 10(3): 263–273.

Berger, T.J., Ander, D.S., Terrell, M.L. & Berle, D.C. (2004). The impact of the demand for clinical productivity on student teaching in academic emergency departments. *Academic Emergency Medicine*, 11(12): 1364–1367.

Driscoll, J. (2006). *Practising clinical supervision: A reflective approach* (2nd ed.). Edinburgh: Bailliere Tindall.

Glicken, A.D. & Merenstein, G.B. (2007). Addressing the hidden curriculum: Understanding educator professionalism. *Medical Teacher*, 29(1): 54–57.

Grossman, S.C. (2007). *Mentoring in nursing: A dynamic and collaborative process*. New York: Springer.

Hays, R. (2007). Developing as a health professional educator: Pathways and choices. *The Clinical Teacher*, 4(1): 46–50.

Heddle, D.O., Himburg, S.P., Collins, N. & Lewis, R. (2002). The professional development portfolio process: Setting goals for credentialing. *Journal of the American Dietetic Association*, 102(10): 1439–1444.

Hoffman, K.G. & Donaldson, J.F. (2004). Contextual tensions of the clinical environment and their influence on teaching and learning. *Medical Education*, 38(4): 448–454.

Johns, C. (2004). *Becoming a reflective practitioner* (2nd ed.). Oxford: Blackwell Publishing.

Johns, C. (2010). *Guided reflection: A narrative approach to advancing professional practice*. West Sussex, UK: Blackwell Publishing.

Kertis, M. (2007). The one-minute preceptor: A five-step tool to improve clinical teaching skills. *Journal for Nurses in Staff Development*, 23(5): 238–242.

Lau, A.K.L., Chuk, K.C. & So, W.K.W. (2002). Reflective practise in clinical teaching. *Nursing and Health Sciences*, 4(4): 201–208.

McKenna, L. (2004). A critical examination of clinical teaching in under-graduate nurse education. Unpublished PhD thesis. Melbourne: Deakin University.

McKimm, J. & Swanwick, T. (2010). *Clinical teaching made easy: A practical guide to teaching and learning in clinical settings.* London: Quay Books.

Megginson, D. & Clutterbuck, D. (2005). *Techniques for coaching and mentoring.* Oxford: Elsevier.

Molodysky, E. (2007). Clinical teacher training: Maximising the 'ad hoc' teaching encounter. *Australian Family Physician*, 36(12): 1044–1046.

Neher, J.O., Gordon, K.C., Meyer, B. & Stevens, N. (1992). A five-step 'microskills' model of clinical teaching. *Journal of the American Board of Family Practice*, 5(4): 419–424.

O'Connor, M. (2011). Beyond the classroom: Nurse-leader preparation and practices. *Nursing Administration Quarterly*, 35(4): 333–337.

Ouellett, M.L. (2007). Your teaching portfolio: Strategies for initiating and documenting growth and development. *Journal of Management Education*, 31(3): 421–433.

Provident, I.M. (2005). Mentoring: A role to facilitate academic change. *The Internet Journal of Allied Health Sciences and Practice*, 3(2).

Raman, S. & Leinster, S. (2008). AMEE guide no. 34: Teaching in the clinical environment. *Medical Teacher*, 30(4): 347–364.

Sambell, K. & McDowell, L. (1998). The construction of the hidden curriculum: Messages and meanings in the assessment of student learning. *Assessment & Evaluation in Higher Education*, 23(4): 391–402.

Schon, D.A. (1983). *The reflective practitioner: How professionals think in action.* New York: Basic Books.

Shafelt, T.D., Oreskovich, M.R., Dyrbye, L.N., Satele, D.V., Hanks, J.B., Sloan, J.A. & Balch, C.M. (2012). Avoiding burnout: The personal health habits and wellness practices of US surgeons. *Annals of Surgery*, 255(4): 625–633.

Steinert, Y. (2005). Staff development for clinical teachers. *The Clinical Teacher*, 2(2): 104–110.

Taylor, B.J. (2010). *Reflective practice for health professionals: A practical guide* (3rd ed.). Maidenhead, UK: Open University Press.

Thiedke, C., Blue, A.V., Chessman, A.W., Keller, A.H. & Mallin, R. (2004). Student observation and ratings of preceptor's interactions with patients: The hidden curriculum. *Teaching and Learning in Medicine: An International Journal*, 16(4): 312–316.

Thistlethwaite, J. (2006). How to keep a portfolio. *The Clinical Teacher*, 3(2): 118–123.

White, S.J. & Tryon, J.E. (2007). How to find and succeed as a mentor. *American Journal of Health-System Pharmacy*, 64(12): 1258–1259.

Xu, Y. (2004). Teacher portfolios: An effective way to assess teacher performance and enhance learning. *Childhood Education*, 80(4): 198–201.

Learning Resource 1
Learning Inventory

Evaluating each individual learner is vital to ensuring optimal learning outcomes. The questions posed in Table LR1.1 provide a checklist by which you can better understand each learner and tailor appropriate learning experiences, thus optimising their learning experiences.

TABLE LR1.1 Learning Inventory Checklist

Learner Characteristics

1. How does the learner prefer to learn?
2. Does the learner have a preferred learning style?
3. What types of teaching and learning best suit the learner?
4. What specific skills does the learner bring to the placement?
5. Are there particular generational factors that need to be considered in planning learning activities?
6. What previous clinical rotations has the learner undertaken, and where have these been done?
7. Does the learner bring with them previous life experiences that might impact on their learning?
8. Does the learner seek to be extended beyond their set learning objectives?
9. Are there any factors that may inhibit clinical learning?

Learner Preparation

10. What is the learner's entry level knowledge and skills base?
11. What academic preparation has the learner had to date?
12. Does the learner demonstrate sufficient knowledge of underlying theory relevant to the types of clients in the setting?
13. What experience has the learner had in simulated practice contexts?
14. Is the learner sufficiently prepared to undertake allocated clinical tasks?
15. What level of complexity does the learner require in practical experiences?
16. Are there cultural aspects that may influence learning effectiveness?

Learning Needs

17. What are the prescribed learning objectives for the experience?
18. What specific competencies does the learner personally seek to achieve during the experience?
19. What preparation does the learner require with regard to the learning environment?

Environmental Factors

20. What are the learner's expectations of the learning environment?
21. What particular aspects of the learning environment will assist learners to meet formal and informal learning objectives?
22. What opportunities does the clinical setting offer to extend the learner's learning?
23. What resources exist to support the learner's particular learning requirements?
24. Are additional resources required to facilitate the achievement of learning outcomes?

Learning Resource 2
Thinking Skills Framework

Constructing meaningful and appropriate learning skills to promote effective thinking can be difficult. Table LR2.1 on pages 234 to 236 provides verbs that can be used in constructing learning outcomes according to the level of thinking required, from the lowest to the highest order.

TABLE LR2.1 Words to Construct Learning Outcomes

Cognitive Domain

LOWER ORDER THINKING SKILLS ——————————————————→ HIGHER ORDER THINKING SKILLS

Remembering	Understanding	Applying	Analysing	Evaluating	Creating
Define	Explain	Apply	Analyse	Appraise	Assess
List	Comprehend	Demonstrate	Illustrate	Contrast	Argue
Record	Discuss	Examine	Compare	Compare	Consider
Label	Generalise	Illustrate	Compute	Critique	Create
Count	Review	Manipulate	Combine	Estimate	Judge
State	Restate	Operate	Compose	Debate	Validate
Name	Tell	Prepare	Discriminate	Defend	Plan
Describe	Estimate	Change	Design	Evaluate	Reconstruct
Repeat	Give examples	Dramatise	Formulate	Estimate	Generate
Underline	Report	Collect	Modify	Interpret	Compose
Identify	Express	Practise	Plan	Justify	Compile
Know	Translate	Calculate	Infer	Score	Categorise
Recall	Paraphrase	Solve	Reconstruct	Summarise	Design
Reproduce	Summarise	Sketch	Revise	Select	Invent
Locate	Rewrite	Select	Relate	Support	Innovate
Tabulate	Infer	Discover	Manage	Combine	Execute
Memorise	Convert	Use	Integrate	Conclude	Construct
Find	Interpret	Predict	Prescribe	Action	Predict
Write	Translate	Produce	Propose	Prioritise	Reflect
Name	Outline	Arrange	Assemble	Rate	Theorise
		Relate	Order	Recommend	Imagine
		Classify	Differentiate	Decide	Hypothesise
		Clarify	Investigate	Monitor	
		Show			

TABLE LR2.1 Words to Construct Learning Outcomes (page 2 of 3)

Affective Domain

DEVELOPING AWARENESS ────────────────────────────────► INTERNALISED VALUES

Receiving	Responding	Valuing	Organisation and Conceptualisation	Characterisation by Value
Ask	Accept	Explain	Alter	Internalise
Focus	Choose	Accept	Arrange	Endure
Follow	Complete	Justify	Discriminate	Discriminate
Accept	Discuss	Complete	Display	Revise
Recognise	Examine	Influence	Judge	Change
Attend	Respond	Prefer	Integrate	Question
Realise	Select	Pursue	Modify	
Listen	Present	Initiate	Organise	
Follow	Answer	Select	Resolve	
Observe	Agree	Follow	Adhere	
Reply	Comply	Ask	Commit	
Develop	Obey	Share	Complete	
	Display	Seek	Defend	
		Value	Combine	
			Order	
			Organise	

(Continues)

TABLE LR2.1 Words to Construct Learning Outcomes (page 3 of 3)

Psychomotor Domain

SIMPLE/EXPOSURE ⟶ COMPLEX/INTERNALISED MASTERY

Perception/ Observation	Guided Responses/ Imitation	Mechanisms/ Precision	Complex Response	Adaptation	Origination
Hear	Copy	Build	Calibrate	Adapt	Construct
See	Assemble	Illustrate	Test	Alter	Create
Smell	Demonstrate	Mix	Reassemble	Change	Design
Taste	Follow	Manipulate	Maintain	Correct	Originate
Touch	Discover	Organise	Operate	Design	Produce
Detect	Duplicate	Discriminate	Demonstrate	Modify	Revise
Separate	Determine	Prepare	Co-ordinate	Build	Arrange
Select	Imitate	Dismantle		Develop	Form
Distinguish	Repeat			Revise	Generate
Locate	Manipulate			Substitute	Craft
Move	Stimulate			Solve	Fashion
React	Display			Shift	
Answer	Apply				
	Adjust				
	React				
	Reproduce				
	Adjust				
	Position				

References

Anderson, L.W. & Krathwohl, D.R. (Eds). (2001). *A taxonomy for learning, teaching, and assessing: A revision of Bloom's taxonomy of educational objectives.* New York: Longman.

Bloom, B.S. & Krathwohl, D.R. (1956). *Taxonomy of educational objectives: The classification of educational goals.* Handbook I: Cognitive domain. New York: Longmans, Green.

Dave, R.H. (1975). Psychomotor levels. In R.J. Armstrong (Ed.), *Developing and writing behavioural objectives.* Tucson, AZ: Educational Innovators Press.

Ferris, T.L.J. (2010). Bloom's taxonomy of educational objectives: A psychomotor skills extension for engineering education. *International Journal of Engineering Education,* 26(3): 699–707.

Ferris, T.L.J. (2011). Bloom's affective domain in systems engineering education. Conference proceedings. Fifth Asia Pacific Council on Systems Engineering (APCOSE), 19–21 October 2011, Seoul, South Korea.

Ferris, T.L.J. & Aziz, S.M. (2005). Psychomotor skills extension to Bloom's taxonomy of education objectives for engineering education. Conference proceedings. Exploring Innovation in Education and Research, Tainan, Taiwan, 1 March 2005.

Krawthwohl, D.R., Bloom, B.S. & Masia, B.B. (1973). *Taxonomy of educational objectives: The classification of educational goals.* Handbook II: Affective domain. New York: David McKay Co. Inc.

Learning Resource 3
Lesson Plans

Use the following template to develop lesson plans for teaching students and clients. It combines preparation and planning items and includes a tool to use during the session to help keep it on track (Table LR3.1).

Teaching plan for: _____ (*topic area*)

1. Overall session aim
2. Learning needs: long and short term, immediate and later priorities
3. Aids or barriers to learning, prior learning and experience
4. Environmental considerations and preparation required
5. Learning outcomes
6. Standard lesson plan (see Table LR3.1).

TABLE LR3.1 Standard Lesson Plan

Time (Minutes)	Content (Topic and Subtopics)	Activities/ Teaching Approaches	Resources	Evaluation Methods
	Introduction	Discussion, lecture, demonstration, student return demonstration (etc.)	PowerPoint© presentation (etc.)	Specific questions to probe understanding (etc.)
	Subtopic 1			
	Subtopic 2			
	Subtopic 3			
	Conclusion			

Learning Resource 4
Questioning Techniques

As a communication skill, questioning is perhaps one of the most complicated. Effective questioning can probe learners' understanding and promote critical thinking. There are numerous reasons for asking questions, such as to:

- Seek information and viewpoints
- Clarify issues
- Challenge accuracy
- Elicit rationale for points of view
- Explore understanding
- Test knowledge
- Expand deeper understandings, implications and consequences
- Seek connections
- Re-orientate or focus attention on key aspects
- Avoid misunderstandings
- Encourage sharing of factual information and feelings
- Lead the respondent to identify problem-solving options
- Build relationships
- Gather information to understand the learners' perceptions more fully
- Sensitively interrogate the learner's depth of knowledge.

Open and Closed Questions

Most questions are formed in response to the circumstances in which they are asked. Questions are often classified as either opened or closed. The opening word is a strong determiner of the degree of openness of the question.

Common words to start closed questions usually include:

- Is/Are
- Have/Does
- Do/Did/Does
- Has/Have
- Can.

Often *closed questions* elicit a response of only 'Yes' or 'No'. These types of questions leave little room for the learner to answer otherwise. However, *open questions* provide greater liberty for the learner to elaborate on their response. Through questioning, we seek to reveal the learners' understanding across four dimensions of knowledge: factual, conceptual, procedural and metacognitive. These are covered in the following examples, where the subject of 'Pain' is used to demonstrate questioning techniques because it is a generic concept for most health professionals.

How: Processes

- How long has he had the pain?
- How frequently is he experiencing the pain?
- How do you think that is related to what you know about the physiology of pain?
- How might you explain any deviations from the normal?
- How might the client's medications affect his ability to manage this daily routine?
- Given what you now know about the client, *how* will you develop an intervention/management/rehabilitation plan for the client?
- How will you involve the client, family and other health professionals in this plan?
- How could you confirm or refute that …?
- How often will he require a review of this pain management schedule?

- How do you know this …?
- How does … affect …?
- How does that relate to what you know about …?
- How could you now look at … differently?
- How did you make this decision?
- How does that compare with what you said before?
- How is what you are saying related to …?

When: Time

- When did he last experience the pain?
- When do you think there should be indication of improvement or adjustment?
- When would you anticipate implementing such a plan?
- When will you …?
- When are you …?
- When would you … as compared with …?
- Tell me more about a time when you …?

Where: Location

- Where exactly did he experience the pain?
- Where would be the best place for this to occur?
- Where is the pain located?

What: Facts

- What can you tell me about Mr …?
- Knowing what you do about Mr …, what problems (decision, actions or interventions) do you foresee?
- What do you think the pain is related to?
- What does that tell you about theories of pain or pain receptors?
- What exactly do you mean by …?

- What evidence is there to suggest this is an appropriate intervention?
- Then what would happen?
- What would happen if ...?
- On what evidence are you basing that?
- What if you compare ... with ...?
- What was significant about ...?
- What physiological response is occurring when ...?
- What else could you confirm/assume from the tests?
- What other strategies does the literature suggest?
- What led you to that decision?
- What will this tell/suggest to you?

Why: Explanations

- Why is he experiencing the pain only when he moves?
- Why do you think that is happening?
- Why is it necessary to ...?
- Why is it important?
- Why is it better than ...?
- Why do you think I asked you that?
- Why do you think that?
- Why did that occur instead of ...?

Would/could

- Could you describe ...?
- Could you tell me what the client says the pain feels like?
- Would that be the first thing you would do, and why?
- You said that the client first experienced the pain three days ago, while at work: could the pain be related to any activity being

undertaken at that time? If so, does that alter your management strategy?

- Could you give me an example?
- Could you tell me more about that, please?
- Could you discuss why you decided on that action/intervention/ plan ...?

Who

- In this client's case, who would be the most appropriate health professional to monitor/consult/refer/manage their treatment and why?
- Who would be most affected by ...?

Affective Questions

Affective questions are used for raising awareness and questioning personal, cultural and social values; responding and reacting with integrity; and choosing and expressing values with a commitment and conviction to those choices. They relate to attitudes, values, emotions, appreciation, personal feelings, society and culture.

How: Feelings

- How did that affect you?
- How did the client react to that situation/suggestion?
- How did you feel about that?
- How would the client's psychological state influence ...?
- How did that make you feel?

Would/could: Open focus, decisions, clarification

- Would you like to talk about it?
- I'm unclear on what you are saying. Could you please try to explain it in a different way?

- Could you describe …?
- Could you explain …?

Empathy

- It seems you are rather upset, could you tell me what happened?
- Could you tell me more about how you are feeling?
- I appreciate that you are feeling … Why do you think those feelings have surfaced?

Psychomotor: Procedural

Learning: Recall

- Tell me what you know about …?
- How would you plan for …?

Application

- Can you show me how you will demonstrate/manipulate/show Mr …?
- Where will you put it?
- Would you put that there?
- Is that the best way to assist the client?
- What educational strategy would you use?

Retention

- How will this influence your behaviour in the future?
- Would you do it the same next time?
- From your interactions with the client, what does your experience now tell you about clients in pain?

Increased Diversity

- How could you do that in the client's home/workplace?
- What other situations might you find you could do …?

- What if the client was a different age? Would that change what you would do?

Motivation and Reinforcement

- You carried out that assessment exceptionally well. What do you think it has taught you?
- That's right! Now what do you think may have influenced/changed/challenged/helped …?

Social

- Tell me why it is important to know how the client will be able to manage at home?
- What do you think might influence his ability to manage?
- How will you know that the services/treatment/interventions are appropriate?

Cultural

- Tell me why you think the client's cultural background may influence his treatment strategy/ability to cope?
- How does the client's culture related to … make a difference to or impact on the outcome?
- Can you tell me how the client's cultural heritage may have a bearing on his attitudes towards …?
- How will you ensure that the client's cultural beliefs are taken into account?

Assessment and Reflection

- Tell me what you thought of …?
- What considerations would you take into account in the future?

- What went well for you as you …?
- Can you tell me how you might do that differently next time?
- How has this experience influenced how you now think about …?
- Tell me how you have achieved your goals?

Reference

Anderson, L.W., Krathwohl, D.R., Airasian, P.W., Cruikshank, K.A., Mayer, R.E. & Pintrich, P.R. (Eds). (2001). *A taxonomy of learning, teaching and assessment: A revision of Bloom's taxonomy of educational objectives*. New York: Longman.

Learning Resource 5
Framework for Reflective Practice

Reflection is central to effective learning and behaviour change. Teachers play an important role in assisting learners to reflect. As a teacher, you also should engage in regular reflection. The following parts can be applied to help achieve this.

Part 1: Describing the Experience

In your own words, provide a detailed description of the experience/event/incident as it unfolded. Consider the following questions:

- What was significant about the event?
- What was challenging about the event?
- Why has it stuck in my memory?
- When did the event take place?
- What went well during the event?
- What caused consternation?
- What essential factors contributed to the event?
- Who were the significant people involved in the event (yourself, the client, team members or significant others)? What was their role or responsibility that influenced the event?
- What reactions of others involved in the event did I notice?
- What was I trying to achieve?
- What were the consequences of my actions for myself, the client, significant others, or those with whom I work?
- How did I feel about the event at the time it happened?

Reflective questions for a team's experience may include:

- What is a description of the event from the perspective of each team member?

- Did we work as a team? If so, what worked well or what can we improve?
- What were the reaffirming and challenging aspects of the interactions during the event/situation?
- How did interactions with others in the team make me feel?
- How do other team members feel about the experience?

Influencing Factors

Consider the influence of feelings, attitudes, beliefs and values:

- What personal factors influenced how the event transpired and my decision making? To what extent did I act for the best and in tune with my values?

Consider where the event took place (the client's home, the clinic or hospital), and organisational factors such as policies. For example:

- What contextual factors influenced the event and my decisions?
- What sources of knowledge (legal, professional, ethical, biosciences) influenced the event and my decisions?
- How may cultural aspects of the event have influenced my actions and decision making?

Consider also historical, economic, political, linguistic factors, patterns of communication, and religious, social, educational, environmental and gender factors.

Reflective questions for a team's influences may include:

- What outstanding or unique contributions did my profession make to this event/situation as part of the team?
- What are the roles of other members of the (healthcare) team, and how important are those roles in this situation/event?
- What are the commonalities/differences between us?
- How do I feel about others' roles and their importance?
- What can I learn from other members of the team of (healthcare) professionals?

Review of Alternative Actions

- What were the general implications of this event to my practices?
- What other choices did I have?
- What other courses of action could I have taken?
- What would have been the intended and unintentional consequences of those choices?
- What factors might constrain me from responding differently?
- How will I know that I have gained knowledge, skills or insights from this event?
- What evidence can I offer to demonstrate that learning has occurred?

Part 2: Outcomes of Reflection

Questions that will indicate outcomes can include:

- How do I now feel about the event?
- Have I learned anything new about myself, the client, others, the situation?
- Has it changed my way of thinking in any way?
- What other knowledge—theories, concepts and research— could have been applied to this situation or event? How do I now incorporate this into my practice?
- Have I been able to confirm or refute my understanding of the event and influencing factors?
- How competent do I now feel to perform/be involved in similar circumstances?
- Considering the influencing factors above, what do I now think of these broader issues? And how will this influence my future practice?
- What insights have I gained?
- How can I use my strengths to address my limitations?

- How has the overall experience and my reflection on it added to my knowledge and competence for future practice?
- How will my learning from this situation or event help improve the quality of client care in the future?

Reflective questions for a team's outcomes are:

- How can I be more receptive to the perspective of other team members?
- How can I promote the inclusion of all team members?
- What can we learn together?
- What can we do together?

Action Plan

- How has this reflective process transformed and/or enriched my knowledge and insights?
- What do I now need to do to further develop my knowledge base or insight, should a similar situation occur in the future?

References

Johns, C. (1994). Guided reflection. In A. Palmer, S. Burns & C. Bulman (Eds). *Reflective practice in nursing*. Oxford: Blackwell Scientific.

Johns, C. (2009). *Becoming a reflective practitioner* (3rd ed.). Oxford: Wiley-Blackwell.

Johns, C. (Ed.). (2010). *Guided reflection: A narrative approach to advancing professional practice* (2nd ed.). Hoboken, NJ: Wiley-Blackwell.

Stockhausen, L. (2007). Developing culturally competent reflective practitioners. Part 1: Cultural reflections. *Asian Journal of Nursing*, 10(4): 212–217.

Stockhausen, L. & Kawashima, A. (2008). Developing culturally competent reflective practitioners. Part 2: A culturally sensitive reflective practice model. *Asian Journal of Nursing*, 11(1): 8–12.

Zarezadeh, Y., Pearson, P. & Dickinson, C. (2009). A model for using reflection to enhance interprofessional education. *International Journal of Education*, 1(1): e12.

Learning Resource 6
Using Evidence

Using evidence effectively is important in health professional education. Educators must use evidence to support their teaching approaches, as well as assist students to use evidence to support their practice. Using evidence ensures that implemented practice and teaching approaches are supported by research. Table LR6.1 provides a basic framework for incorporating evidence into teaching and clinical practice.

TABLE LR6.1 Evidence Framework

Stage 1	**Develop a question that can be answered** The question should address a particular need or problem. This may be around a particular clinical problem or teaching situation. (See the following pages to structure questions of clinical inquiry and relevance using PICOT [Sackett, et al. 2000; Melnyk, et al. 2010].)	CASE EXAMPLE *A teacher wants to know how to assist students to deal with the death of a patient. He develops the question 'What are students' reactions to death and dying, and how can they be assisted to deal with the situations?'*
Stage 2	**Search for best evidence** Online databases provide access to large amounts of research evidence to inform teaching and practice. Some relevant sources include: • Health or medical databases such as CINAHL, Medline, PsycINFO, Cochrane Library, Joanna Briggs • Education portals such as ERIC • Searches within the databases developed from key words that clearly reflect the problem area.	*Using key words 'teaching', 'student' and 'death' in CINAHL and Medline, the teacher sources 48 articles meeting the search criteria. These include articles about how students' cope with death and dying, as well as strategies for dealing with such events.*

TABLE LR6.1 Evidence Framework (*continued*)

Stage 3	**Appraise evidence sourced** In appraising the evidence, key questions need to be asked: • What is the overall quality of the study? • Are the findings valid; that is, is there any bias in the results? • Did the study test what it set out to test? • Do the results support the conclusions drawn? • Are the results obtained able to be implemented; that is, can they be generalised to populations beyond those studied?	*After selecting key articles from those sourced, the teacher evaluates the types of studies undertaken, assesses their validity, and identifies one approach for supporting his students in practice.*
Stage 4	**Apply the evidence** If valid evidence is located, it can then be put into practice.	*The chosen approach to supporting students is put into practice.*
Stage 5	**Evaluating the use of the evidence** Finally, once the evidence has been applied to practice, it needs to be evaluated in the context in which it was applied.	*The implementation of the approach is evaluated, and modified if needed. At this stage, it might be decided that returning to the evidence is required. The teacher chooses to evaluate his approach with feedback from students and other health professionals, as well as observing students' coping skills.*

Adapted from Sackett, D.L., Richardson, W.S., Rosenberg, W.M. et al. (2000). *Evidence-based medicine: How to practice and teach EBM* (2nd ed.). Edinburgh: Churchill Livingstone.

Steps to Develop PICOT

Steps in developing PICO(T) questions to structure an evidence-based practice (EBP) investigation (Sackett et al., 2000; Melnyk & Fineout-Overholt, 2011; Melnyk et al., 2010; Facchiano & Snyder, 2012a, 2012b) and cultivate a spirit of enquiry, are as follows:

1. Ask the clinical question in the PICOT format:
   - **P: Population/disease:** age, gender, ethnicity, with a certain disorder
   - **I: Intervention** or Variable of Interest: exposure to a disease, risk behaviour, possibilities, prognostic factor
   - **C: Comparison**: could be a placebo or as presently practiced
   - **O: Outcome:** risk of disease, accuracy of a diagnosis, rate of occurrence or adverse outcome
   - **T: Time:** unit of time it takes to demonstrate an outcome (e.g. the time it takes for the intervention to achieve an outcome or how long participants are observed).

   Note: Not every question will have an intervention (as in a meaning question) or time aspect (when it is implied in another part of the question).

2. Search for and collect the most relevant best evidence (see Table LR6.2).

TABLE LR6.2 Best Type of Evidence for Your Question

Type of Question	Ideal Type of Evidence to Search For (or add as a key search word)
Intervention	1. Systematic reviews/meta-analysis (synthesis) of Randomised Controlled Trials (RCTs)
	2. RCTs
	3. Non-randomised controlled trials
	4. Cohort study or case-control studies
	5. Meta-synthesis of qualitative or descriptive studies
	6. Qualitative or descriptive studies
	7. Expert opinions

TABLE LR6.2 Best Type of Evidence for Your Question (*continued*)

Type of Question	Ideal Type of Evidence to Search For (or add as a key search word)
Diagnosis or diagnostic test Prognosis/ prediction	1. Synthesis of cohort study or case-control studies 2. Single cohort study or case-control studies 3. Meta-synthesis of qualitative or descriptive studies 4. Single qualitative or descriptive studies 5. Expert opinion
Aetiology Meaning	1. Meta-synthesis of qualitative studies 2. Single qualitative studies 3. Synthesis of descriptive studies 4. Single descriptive studies 5. Expert opinions

3. Critically appraise the evidence using the hierarchy suggested in Table LR6.3.

TABLE LR6.3 Rating System for the Hierarchy of Evidence for Intervention/Treatment Questions

Level	Source of Evidence
I	Systematic review or meta-analysis of all relevant RCTs
II	Well-designed RCTs
III	Well-designed controlled trials without randomisation
IV	Well-designed case-control and cohort studies
V	Reviews of descriptive and qualitative studies
VI	Single descriptive or qualitative studies
VII	Opinion of authorities and/or reports of expert committees

4. Integrate the best evidence with one's clinical expertise, client preferences and values in making a practice decision or change.
5. Evaluate outcomes of the practice decision or change based on evidence.
6. Disseminate the outcomes of the EBP decision or change.

Sample Questions using PICOT

Some example templates for posing clinical questions using PICOT (Melnyk & Fineout-Overholt, 2011, p. 31) are given in Table LR6.4.

TABLE LR6.4 Sample PICOT Questions

Intervention/Therapy

In _____ (P), what is the effect of _____ (I) on _____ (O) compared with _____ (C) within _____ (T)?

In _____ (P), how does _____ (I) compared with _____ (C) affect _____ (O) within _____ (T)?

Aetiology

Are _____ (P) who have _____ (I) at _____ (increased/decreased) risk for/of _____ (O) compared with _____ (P) with/without _____ (C) over _____ (T)?

Diagnosis or Diagnostic Test

Are (is) _____ (I) more accurate in diagnosing _____ (P) compared with _____ (C) for _____ (O)?

In _____ (P), are/is _____ (I) compared with _____ (C) more accurate in diagnosing _____ (O)?

Prevention

For _____ (P), does the use of _____ (I) reduce the future risk of _____ (O) compared with _____ (C)?

Prognosis/Predictions

Does _____ (I) influence _____ (O) in patients who have _____ (P) over _____ (T)?

Meaning

How do _____ (P) diagnosed with _____ (I) perceive _____ (O) during _____ (T)?

Etiology/Causation

Are _____ (P) who have _____ (I) compared with those without _____ (C) at _____ risk for/of _____ (O) over _____ (T)?

References and Further Reading

American Psychological Association. (2011). PsycINFO. Retrieved November 2012 from www.apa.org/pubs/databases/psycinfo/index.aspx.

Bandolier: Evidence-Based Thinking about Healthcare. (2011). About Bandolier and us. Retrieved November 2012 at www.medicine.ox.ac.uk/bandolier/aboutus.html.

Baumann, S. (2010). The limitations of evidenced-based practice. *Nursing Science Quarterly*, 23(3): 226–230.

Elkins, M. (2010). Using PICO and the brief report to answer clinical questions. *Nursing*, 40(4): 59–60.

Facchiano, L. & Snyder, C. (2012a). Evidence-based practice for the busy nurse practitioner. Part one: Relevance to clinical practice and clinical inquiry process. *Journal of the American Academy of Nurse Practitioners*, 24(10): 579–586.

Facchiano, L. & Snyder, C. (2012b). Evidence-based practice for the busy nurse practitioner. Part two: Searching for the best evidence to clinical inquiries. *Journal of the American Academy of Nurse Practitioners*, 24(11): 640–648.

Fineout-Overholt, E., Melnyk, B., Stillwell, S. & Williamson, K. (2010). Evidence-based practice step by step: Critical appraisal of the evidence. Part I. *American Journal of Nursing*, 110(7): 47–52.

Melnyk, B. & Fineout-Overholt, E. (2011). *Evidence-based practice in nursing and healthcare: A guide to best practice* (2nd ed.). Philadelphia, PA: Wolters Kluwer Health/Lippincott Williams & Wilkins.

Melnyk, B., Fineout-Overholt, E., Stillwell, S. & Williamson, K. (2010). Evidence-based practice: Step by step. The seven steps of evidence-based practice. *American Journal of Nursing*, 110(1): 51–53.

Sackett, D.L., Richardson, W.S., Rosenberg, W.M. et al. (2000). *Evidence-based medicine: How to practice and teach EBM* (2nd ed.). Edinburgh: Churchill Livingstone.

Straus, S., Glasizou, P., Richardson, W. & Haynes, R. (2011). Evidence-based medicine: How to practice and teach it (4th ed.). Edinburgh London: Churchill Livingstone Elsevier.

The Cochrane Library. (2011). Independent high quality evidence for health care decision making. Retrieved November 2012 at www.thecochranelibrary.com/view/0/AboutTheCochraneLibrary.html.

Worral, P., Levin, R. & Côté-Arsenault, D. (2009). Documenting an EBP project: Guidelines for what to include and why. *Journal of the New York State Nurses Association*, 40(2): 12–19.

Learning Resource 7
Teaching Evaluation

Students often perform formal evaluations of classroom teaching. However, if you are teaching in the practice setting, consider asking your peers or university staff to provide an evaluation of your performance, too, if one is not routinely performed. A variety of tools exist for evaluating teaching in practice settings. The tool in Table LR7.1 provides questions that you may tailor to evaluate your teaching, and the results can be included in your teaching portfolio.

TABLE LR 7.1 Teaching Evaluation Tool

Criteria	Never	Seldom	Sometimes	Usually	Always
Professional Practice Develops constructive relationships in the teaching/learning setting					
Acts as a professional role model					
Demonstrates and promotes empathy in interactions with clients and families					
Practices in accordance with professional codes					
Feedback Encourages learners to provide feedback					
Provides individualised, constructive feedback on student performance					
Provides timely feedback on student performance					
Teaching Encourages application of classroom theory to practice					

TABLE LR 7.1 Teaching Evaluation Tool (*continued*)

Criteria	Never	Seldom	Sometimes	Usually	Always
Teaching Promotes reflective learning					
Encourages critical thinking and problem solving					
Provides opportunities for students to reflect and debrief on their learning					
Enables learners to achieve learning objectives					
Supports learners in challenging situations					
Provides clear directions and demonstrations					
Asks questions that extend learning and reflection					
Provides sufficient time for teaching and learning					
Provides opportunities for students to meet required learning objectives					
Responds promptly to questions and concerns					
Stimulates students to learn more					
Encourages hands-on practice					
Identifies teaching and learning resources in the particular setting					
Implements evidence-based approaches to teaching and clinical practice					

Note: Extended-response feedback could include:
• Aspects you did well
• Aspects you could develop further
• Effectiveness of your interaction
• Aspects of your teaching style.

Learning Resource 8
Learning Environment Evaluation

According to Health Workforce Australia (2011, p. 7), 'Clinical placements should facilitate education and learning in a safe, supportive and appropriately resourced work environment'. Knowledge of the local environment alerts the teacher to idiosyncrasies that influence the learning environment, inclusive of safety, support and resources. Often it is not until we are asked to reflect on it that we are alerted to the environment's influence on learning and teaching.

The following questions incorporate a range of research (Bloomfield & Subramaniam, 2008; Chan, 2002; Fraser et al. 1987; Moos, 1980; 1994a; 1994b; Moos & Trickett, 1987; Rogers, 2001) and were developed to evaluate the learning environment; in particular, the clinical learning environment. Responses to the questions will alert the teacher as to where further communication or developments are required to prepare the environment for learners and for themselves.

The reference list provides a comprehensive array of both classroom and clinical learning environment resources and tools that may be accessed by the teacher for further intensive investigation and application.

Environment

- What is the locality of the organisation?
- Can learners adequately access the facility?
- Are arrangements in place that will physically accommodate the learners?
- What is the general layout of the physical environment/s?
- How does the layout impact on the interactions that are required to take place and on the type of work carried out?
- Are there any physical variables of the environment (smells, noise level, lighting, heating, cooling, ventilation, building/room or clinic layout) related to work efficiency, comfort or interactions,

which impact on the fulfilment of role requirements and/or the care or treatment of clients?

- What type of health professionals occupy the space; for example, radiographers, physiotherapists, pharmacists, nurses, social workers?
- What is unique about this particular field?
- Do learners have the opportunity for interprofessional interaction and learning opportunities?
- How does the organisation value learning and learners and provide opportunities for ongoing learning? How are they made visible?
- Are there physical resources to support learning; for example, breakout rooms, Internet/Intranet access?
- What other learning resources are available?
- Is there a detailed orientation for learners?
- What emergency procedures (such as occupational workplace health and safety, fire and resuscitation) do learners need to be aware of?
- How are aspects of the physical and extended environment made visible to the learner (e.g. historical, social, political aspects, economic issues, sustainability practices)?
- How do these aspects influence or impact on the client and/or the practice area, the learner, staff and teacher?

People

- How are staff members prepared for the learner?
- What type of health service users (clients) does the practice area cater for (e.g. ages, conditions, situations, interventions, treatments)?
- What are the staff profiles, demographics, structure and roles in the practice area?

- What are the professional and academic qualifications of staff to support learners?
- Are there opportunities for staff development?
- Does the practice area reflect respect for the rights of health service users, careers, staff and learners? How is this made visible?
- How are service users engaged in their care or treatment?
- Are there sufficient staff members to facilitate and observe learners' requirements and development?
- Are opportunities created for all personnel involved in learners' experiences to provide and receive feedback?

Climate

- What is the overall organisational structure and channels of communication?
- How are all aspects of the organisation involved in the learner's experience?
- What are the organisational and practice area's philosophy and approach to care and treatments?
- Is there evidence of the application of theory and research to care and treatments?
- Is there a good group dynamic and support for one another in the practice setting? How is this determined?
- Are staff members considered approachable? How would you determine this?
- Do staff members have a commitment to learners? How would you determine this?

Learner Engagement

- What role do you and other staff in your practice area consider learners play during their learning experiences?

- What activities do you, and other staff, encourage learners to engage with in the practice area?
- Do learners receive an appropriate level of supervision and support for their level of ability? How is this determined?
- How are learners' individualised plans for their learning incorporated into the everyday practices of the setting? How are opportunities identified/negotiated for the learner to achieve competencies?
- How are learner activities planned? And by whom?
- How are learning opportunities created to develop: knowledge integration; skill acquisition and competencies; and the use of research as a base for practice? How do you identify learning opportunities?
- How are interesting and productive experiences, teaching techniques, learning activities and patient/client allocations implemented for learners?
- How are students' decision making and opportunities for independence identified and supported?
- What is the involvement of the learner in interprofessional engagement and teamwork?
- Are learners' needs, achievements and opportunities reviewed regularly? And by whom?
- How are learners assessed? Are there appropriate and qualified staff members to assess learners?
- How are learners given the opportunity to self-assess?
- What processes are in place for learners to feel safe to raise issues of concern with the teacher or clinical staff?

References and Further Resources

Allodi, M. (2010). The meaning of social climate of learning environments: Some reasons why we do not care enough about it. *Learning Environments Research*, 13(2): 89–104.

Bloomfield, L. & Subramaniam, R. (2008). Development of an instrument to measure the clinical learning environment in diagnostic radiology. *Journal of Medical Imaging and Radiation Oncology*, 52(3): 262–268.

Brown, T., Williams, B., McKenna, L., Palermo, C., McCall, L., Roller, L., Hewitt, L., Molloy, L., Baird, M. & Aldabah, L. (2011). Practice education learning environments: The mismatch between perceived and preferred expectations of undergraduate health science students. *Nurse Education Today*, 31(9): e22–e28.

Chan, D. (2001). Development of an innovative tool to assess hospital learning environments. *Nurse Education Today*, 21(8): 624–631.

Chan, D. (2002). Development of the clinical learning environment inventory: Using the theoretical framework of learning environment studies to assess nursing students' perceptions of the hospital as a learning environment. *Journal of Nursing Education*, 41(2): 69–75.

Chan, D. & Ip, W.Y. (2007). Perception of hospital learning environment: A survey of Hong Kong nursing students. *Nurse Education Today*, 27(7): 677–684.

Chan, D.S. (2002). Associations between student learning outcomes from their clinical placement and their perceptions of the social climate of the clinical learning environment. *International Journal of Nursing Studies*, 39(5): 517–524.

Chan, D.S. (2003). Validation of the clinical learning environment inventory. *Western Journal of Nursing Research*, 25(5): 519–532.

Chan, D.S. (2004). Nursing students' perception of hospital learning environments: An Australian perspective. *International Journal of Nursing Education Scholarship*, 1(1): 1–13.

Chan, D.S. (2004). The relationship between student learning outcomes from their clinical placement and their perceptions of the social climate of the clinical learning environment. *Contemporary Nurse*, 17(1–2): 149–158.

Fraser, B., Treagust, D., Williamson, J. & Tobin, K. (1987). Validation and application of the College & University Classroom Environment Inventory (CUCEI). In B.J. Fraser (Ed.), *The study of learning environments* (pp. 17–30). Perth, WA: Curtin University of Technology.

Health Workforce Australia. (2011). *National clinical supervision support framework*. Adelaide: Health Workforce Australia.

Henderson, A., Heel, A., Twentyman, M & Lloyd, B. (2006). Students' perception of the psycho-social clinical learning environment: an evaluation of placement models. *Nurse Education Today*, 26(7): 564–571.

Moos, R. (1994a). *The social climate scales: A users' guide* (2nd ed.). Palo Alto, CA: Consulting Psychologists Press.

Moos, R. (1994b). *Work environment scale manual: Development, application, research* (3rd ed.). Palo Alto, CA: Consulting Psychologists Press.

Moos, R.H. (1974). *The social climate scales: An overview.* Palo Alto, CA: Consulting Psychologists Press.

Moos, R.H. (1980). Evaluating classroom learning environments. *Studies in Educational Evaluation*, 6: 239–252.

Moos, R.H. & Trickett, E.J. (1987). *Classroom environment scale manual* (2nd ed.). Palo Alto, CA: Consulting Psychologists Press.

Rogers, J. (2001). *Placements in focus: Guidance for education in practice for health professionals.* English National Board for Nursing, Midwifery and Health Visitors and Department of Health. Luton: Chiltern Press.

Saarikoski, M., Isoaho, H., Warne, T. & Leino-Kilpi, H. (2008). The nurse teacher in clinical practice: Developing the new subdimension to the clinical learning environment and supervision (CLES) scale. *International Journal of Nursing Studies*, 45(8): 1233–1237.

Smedley, A. & Morey, P. (2010). Improving learning in the clinical nursing environment: Perceptions of senior Australian bachelor of nursing students. *Journal of Research in Nursing*, 15(1): 75–88.

Index